SpringerBriefs in Criminology

SpringerBriefs in Policing

Series Editor
M. R. Haberfeld
City University of New York
John Jay College of Criminal Justice
New York, NY, USA

SpringerBriefs in Policing presents concise summaries of cutting edge research in Police Science, across the fields of Criminology, Criminal Justice, Psychology, Forensic Science, and Corrections with implications for the study of police and police work. It publishes small but impactful volumes of between 50–125 pages, with a clearly defined focus. The series covers a broad range of Policing research: from experimental design and methods, to brief reports and regional case studies, to policy-related applications.

The scope of the series spans the subfield of Policing, with an aim to be on the leading edge and continue to advance research. The series is international and crossdisciplinary, including a broad array of topics. The main goal of the series is to present innovations in Policing, in order to further the field as a research and evidence-based profession rather than a vocational occupation. It will showcase how Policing confronts problems and challenges that transcend cultures and borders and can be addressed from a global rather than local perspective.

SpringerBriefs in Policing is aimed at a broad range of researchers and practitioners working in Criminology and Criminal Justice Research and in related academic fields such as Public Policy, Sociology, Psychology, Public Health, Economics, Policy Analysis, Terrorism and Political Science.

More information about this series at https://link.springer.com/bookseries/11179

Laura Huey • Jennifer L. Schulenberg
Jacek Koziarski

Policing Mental Health

Public safety and crime prevention in Canada

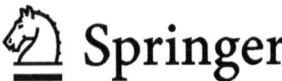

Laura Huey
Department of Sociology
University of Western Ontario
London, ON, Canada

Jennifer L. Schulenberg
Department of Sociology and Legal Studies
University of Waterloo
Waterloo, ON, Canada

Jacek Koziarski
Department of Sociology
University of Western Ontario
London, ON, Canada

ISSN 2192-8533 ISSN 2192-8541 (electronic)
SpringerBriefs in Criminology
ISSN 2194-6213 ISSN 2194-6221 (electronic)
SpringerBriefs in Policing
ISBN 978-3-030-94312-7 ISBN 978-3-030-94313-4 (eBook)
https://doi.org/10.1007/978-3-030-94313-4

© The Author(s), under exclusive license to Springer Nature Switzerland AG 2022
This work is subject to copyright. All rights are solely and exclusively licensed by the Publisher, whether the whole or part of the material is concerned, specifically the rights of translation, reprinting, reuse of illustrations, recitation, broadcasting, reproduction on microfilms or in any other physical way, and transmission or information storage and retrieval, electronic adaptation, computer software, or by similar or dissimilar methodology now known or hereafter developed.
The use of general descriptive names, registered names, trademarks, service marks, etc. in this publication does not imply, even in the absence of a specific statement, that such names are exempt from the relevant protective laws and regulations and therefore free for general use.
The publisher, the authors and the editors are safe to assume that the advice and information in this book are believed to be true and accurate at the date of publication. Neither the publisher nor the authors or the editors give a warranty, expressed or implied, with respect to the material contained herein or for any errors or omissions that may have been made. The publisher remains neutral with regard to jurisdictional claims in published maps and institutional affiliations.

This Springer imprint is published by the registered company Springer Nature Switzerland AG
The registered company address is: Gewerbestrasse 11, 6330 Cham, Switzerland

Preface

In the spring of 2020, the Royal Society of Canada conceived a unique program idea: in response to the Covid-19 virus and its health, social, economic, and other impacts, they would commission a multidisciplinary task force of experts to review evidence and provide information to the public on issues that potentially affect the well-being of Canadians. Taskforce members were asked to convene working groups to produce policy briefs on subjects ranging from economic recovery and vaccine acceptance to health impacts for Indigenous and other racialized communities.

In the fall of 2020, I was asked to join the Taskforce to head up a working group on mental health and policing.[1] Although I was not privy to the discussions that lead to the idea to create this group, undoubtedly media coverage of local protests in the early summer of 2000 in response to police-involved deaths of individuals with mental illness played a role.

Since at least the 1960s, researchers have been documenting the role that police have come to play in the lives of many individuals with mental illness (PMI). Early ethnographies of frontline policing—often conducted in extremely marginalized communities—reveal a complex portrait of these interactions, with police officers frequently acting in what has been termed a form of 'social work' capacity. Under this umbrella of 'social work', we see officers acting as unofficial gatekeepers to mental health resources and/or arresting PMI without stable housing as a means of providing a safe place to stay. In the 1970s and 1980s, much of the research literature in this area became more critical, documenting increasing rates of PMI involvement with the criminal justice system. Throughout the 1990s and 2000s, this critical focus remained; however the work was gradually supplemented with a growing body of research aimed at evaluating programs, policies, and practices aimed at improving police response to the various challenges of responding to the needs of PMI. It was this latter body of evidence which the new working group was tasked

---

[1] The working group is comprised of some of the best Canadian scholars in this area, including Professors Judith Andersen, Craig Bennell, Mary Ann Campbell, and Adam Vaughan. Our efforts were supplemented by those of two amazing early career researchers, Jacek Koziarski and Lorna Ferguson.

with assessing in order to construct what we hoped would be a set of useful policy recommendations.

No policy exercise is completely isolated from the politics of the day. At the time the Policing and Mental Health working group was being formed, a series of calls to 'defund the police' were being heard by groups across the U.S., Canada, the U.K., and elsewhere. As we document in Chapter 1, in Canada the rationale behind these calls was ostensibly that money spent on policing services would be better allocated to 'upstream' preventative solutions or to 'downstream' diversion programs run by mental health and/or social workers. One significant implication of such approaches being that prevention and/or diversion would reduce the volume of police calls for service. As a researcher I never accept something at face value. In part, my skepticism in this instance was based on working experience of police RMS (record management system) and CAD (computer-aided dispatch) data. Poring over thousands of missing persons records had demonstrated to me that many of these 'misspers' calls involve a mental health component that was not captured in how the call codes. If we were to reduce the footprint of policing in relation to calls involving PMI, then we needed to get a better understanding of the data and its limitations. The result was a report, 'The Limits of Our Knowledge: Tracking the Size and Scope of Police Involvement with Persons with Mental Illness', which laid out just how little we know about this subject.[2]

The release of 'The Limits' report, although it shed much needed attention on an important policy issue, was not wholly satisfying. Unanswered questions remained. Among them: how can we better account for the volume and scope of interactions involving police and individuals with mental illness? This book is an attempt to answer that question by drawing on a unique data source: qualitative field notes from two different projects using systematic social observation of frontline policing conducted by my colleague and co-author, Jennifer Schulenberg. With unprecedented access to two different police services, Jenn spent the better part of almost 4 years in and out of patrol cars, observing officers responding to calls for service. In that time, she collected data on approximately 400 encounters between police and citizens.

Our intention in the pages that follow is to sketch out the diverse—and often hidden—ways in which the lives of PMI intersect with policing. We also address the important underlying question of why mental illness has become 'police property'—that is, why policing has too often become the de facto response to a health and social problem, the roots of which lie far outside their ability to prevent or control. As we argue throughout, it is answers to these two inter-related questions that will help inform future policy efforts.

London, ON, Canada
September 3, 2021

Laura Huey

---

[2] These problems with police data are hardly unique to Canada; discussions with policing researchers and crime analysts in the U.S. point to similar problems with relying on police data in many parts of this country.

Contents

1 **Calling the Cops: What Do We Know About the Policing of Individuals with Mental Illness?** 1
   The Concept of 'Police Property' 2
   Police Mobilization 3
   The Disordered and the Disorderly 5
   The Data 6
   The Book 10
   References 11

2 **The Public Safety Role** 15
   Mental Health Apprehensions 15
   Missing Persons 18
   Wellness Checks 19
   Suicide 20
   Follow-up Calls 23
   'Hidden' PMI Calls 23
   Conclusions 24
   References 25

3 **Crime Prevention and Response Role** 27
   Victim-Complainants 28
   PMI as Suspects or Potential Suspects 31
   Conclusions 36
   References 36

4 **Police Attitudes Towards Their Roles in Dealing with Mental Health Issues** 39
   Is Mental Health a Significant Policing Issue? 39
   Should Mental Health Be 'Police Property'? 40
   The Impact of These Calls on Officers 43
   Conclusions 45
   References 46

5	**At the Crossroads**	49
	Upstream Solutions	50
	Downstream Solutions	53
	The Need for Continuous Evaluation	54
	Conclusions	56
	References	56

Appendix: The Studies 59
    Data Collection 59
    Site 1 59
    Site 2 60

References 61

Index 63

Chapter 1
Calling the Cops: What Do We Know About the Policing of Individuals with Mental Illness?

On May 27, 2020, Toronto's emergency dispatch received several calls requesting police presence at a domestic disturbance involving multiple allegations of threats and violence, from punches to knives thrown. When police arrived, along with emergency medical services, one of the complainants requested that her daughter, Regis Korchinski-Paquet, be taken to a mental health facility to de-escalate the situation. While first responders were deliberating as to whether there were grounds to apprehend Ms. Korchinski-Paquet under provincial mental health law, she requested to use the washroom. Once inside, she went onto the balcony of her apartment, holding the door closed to prevent officers from coming out after her. She then tried to climb to a neighbouring balcony, lost her balance, and plummeted 24 stories to her death.

In the early days of this resulting investigation, a number of serious allegations were publicly raised, some police critics even suggesting the police had deliberately thrown Ms. Korchinski-Paquet, a woman of colour, off the balcony. Others questioned whether police actions, or even their mere presence, had escalated the crisis. Most critics—regardless of their beliefs as to the culpability of police in Ms. Korchinski-Paquet's death—argued that police should not be attending calls for service involving mental health crises.

The Korchinski-Paquet case, we argue, is illustrative of some of the complexities surrounding how, when, where, and why police become involved in situations involving persons with mental illness (PMI). It has long been argued that, as a result of chronic underfunding of the social safety net, mental health has become 'police property' (McDaniel, 2019; Wood et al., 2017). Indeed, much has also been written on the role of de-institutionalization, changes in mental health legislation, and the lack of coordinated community services and supports for those with serious mental health disorders (Rogers, 1990; Teplin & Pruett, 1992; Lamb et al., 2002; Coleman & Cotton, 2010; Tribolet-Hardy et al., 2015). This book is focused on a much more specific subset of this topic: what are the different ways in which mental health-related issues have become 'police property'? (Cray, 1972; see also Reiner, 1992).

The Concept of 'Police Property'

Originally coined by Cray (1972) and later refined by Lee (1981, pp. 53–54), the concept of 'police property' refers to when 'the dominant powers of society (in the economy, polity, etc.) leave the problems of [particular groups] to the police'. These groups, as Reiner (1992) elaborates, are low-status and powerless and are commonly perceived as 'problematic' or 'distasteful' by the majority population. The police, in this instance, are expected to deal with this 'property' through means accessible to them, such as law enforcement and order maintenance (ibid.).

There are many examples of 'police property' within modern policing history, and perhaps no example is more relevant to this concept than that of 'skid-row'. As documented extensively elsewhere, 'skid-row' refers to districts found within some urban city-centres in which the so-called problem populations are contained—many of whom are experiencing homelessness, substance use disorder, and/or mental illness—in order to be kept out of sight of populated public spaces (Bittner, 1967; Huey, 2007). Indeed, some cities, such as Los Angeles deliberately created their skid-row districts through explicit policy and urban planning, whereby brightened streetlights and locked trash cans demarcated where skid-row residents do and do no 'belong' (Deener et al., 2013). The containment of skid-row districts and the policing of their residents within, to no surprise, has been left for the police to address. As Bittner (1967) describes this space, patrol officers who are assigned to skid-row are often left to their own devices as to how best deal with the issues found within, whether that be through law enforcement, social work or peacekeeping. Outside skid-row, the police may rely on order maintenance in an effort to re-direct individuals to where their presence is deemed 'acceptable' (Deener et al., 2013; Stuart, 2016).

As can be seen through the 'skid-row' example, police have long been called upon by policy-makers and citizens alike to deal with various behaviours that offend moral sensibilities and are thus recast as socially disruptive and/or harmful to individuals and others. These are the so-called vice crimes. Not surprisingly then, another example of 'police property'—spurred on by the war on drugs—are narcotics and substance use. This drug 'war' effectively sought to aggressively 'crackdown' on those who use drugs through increased policing and mandatory minimum sentencing (Benson et al., 1995; Cooper, 2015; Lynch, 2012). Within this context, those who engage in the 'undesirable' behaviour of drug use were stripped of the opportunity to seek out treatment by instead being classified as 'police property'. This, by consequence, led to an exorbitant number of individuals—who are disproportionately persons of colour—being arrested, charged, and incarcerated for low-level, non-violent drug offences at exponential rates in subsequent decades (Baum, 1997; Cooper, 2015). Furthermore, drug use as 'police property' is multi-faceted in that the police not only partake in the enforcement of drug laws, but also play a role in the (attempted) prevention of drug use as well. Drug Abuse Resistance Education (D.A.R.E., 2021), for example, is a program started in part by the Los Angeles Police Department in the 1980s that seeks to inform students on drug use and its potential consequences. Although the original D.A.R.E. program, and subsequent iterations of it, are still regularly being conducted to this day, numerous studies have found D.A.R.E. to be an ineffective method of lowering drug use (e.g., West & O'Neal, 2004; Rosenbaum, 2007).

Indeed, to a certain extent, many social problems have become 'police property' in one way or another due to the multi-layered nature of the issues that the police are expected to deal with on a daily basis. Even by simply looking at the two provided examples, one can easily point to how the focus of this book—mental health—is already implicated as 'police property' within these closely-related issues. As mentioned, many of those residing on skid-row live with mental illness, whereas in terms of substance use, many studies point to the co-occurrence of mental illness and substance use during interactions between the police and PMI (Charette et al., 2011; Shore & Lavoie, 2019). This book seeks to more fully flesh-out how mental health has become 'police property' within the context of crime and disorder, as well as under the guise of public safety more broadly. In the next section we breakdown the police mandate as it pertains to crime, disorder, and public safety.

Police Mobilization

> ...no human problem exists, or is imaginable, about which it could be said with finality that this certainly could not become the proper business of the police. (Bittner, 1990, p. 250)

Most would, without hesitation, ascribe the detection, investigation, and prevention of crime as a job that the police 'do'. In fact, this role has been part of the police mandate ever since the modern policing institution was conceived under the *Metropolitan Police Act* in 1829 in the United Kingdom (Emsley, 2003). From its inception, the police institution almost solely engaged in what some have labelled as the 'one-size-fits-all' model of policing. Within this model, the police largely placed emphasis on *reacting* to crime that had already occurred (Sherman, 2013; Skogan & Frydl, 2004), even though prevention of crime was also part of the police mandate. Indeed, widespread increases in crime throughout the 1970s and 1980s spurred questions as to whether the police were even capable to prevent crime to begin with and whether crime prevention should be part of the police mandate (Bayley, 1994). The 1990s, however, bore witness to an era of innovation of policing which sought to pivot the institution from the reactive approach toward more effective means of dealing with crime (Weisburd & Braga, 2006). Although, in spite of these developments, responding to crime remains core to the police mandate.

A second aspect of the police mandate is managing disorder, or more broadly: order maintenance. This part of the mandate similarly finds its origins at the conception of the modern police institution (Philips, 1977) and is defined by Wilson (1968, p. 16) as the regulation of behaviour 'that disturbs or threatens to disturb the public peace or that involves face-to-face conflict among two or more persons'. Indeed, what falls under the auspices of 'order maintenance' is far broader than that of crime as it not only encompasses the regulation of social behaviours, such as public drunkenness and public urination, but physical conditions as well, such as graffiti and vandalism (Wilson & Kelling, 1982). Beyond social and physical disorder, order maintenance also involves other matters. More specifically, as Bittner (1990) describes, the police have been positioned within society as the 'or else' option when it comes to conflict resolution:

> The noisy neighbour, the uncooperative tenant, the abusive spouse, the assaultive customer, the unruly youth, the unmanageable patient, and so forth are all the sort of challenges citizens hand over to the police with the expectation that the officer may, can, and will force the recalcitrant into compliance 'then and there' (Bittner, 1990, p. 11).

Within the order maintenance context, the public resorts to—as Bittner (1990) puts it—'calling the cops' to deal with their problems.

However, as the quote presented at the beginning of this section illustrates, the notion of 'calling the cops' is indeed far broader than crime and disorder alone. The police are often put in the position—whether it be through public policy, citizen pressure or other means—to respond to situations which fall under the broader auspices of 'public safety'. As the term may itself suggest, any situation in which the protection or welfare of one or more individuals is of concern, falls under the public safety umbrella. This can range from a vulnerable individual who has been reported missing to a situation in which someone is threatening to take their own life, or even natural or man-made disasters.

One of the complaints frequently heard from police reform groups is that police are 'not social workers'—that is, they lack the skills and training to facilitate or provide social services to individuals in need. And yet, historically, this is the exact role that police have come to play in many instances, serving as informal conduits, or in some instances as formal 'gatekeepers', to resources ranging from mental health to temporary food and shelter (Sellers et al., 2005; Huey, 2007). Bittner's own research in the 1960s documents this role, and the implications of his work were subsequently developed by other field-based researchers who similarly observed that police engaged in a number of activities that had little to do with law enforcement or peacekeeping, from putting runaways on buses home to securing shelter beds for individuals in need (Wiseman, 1970; McSheehy, 1979; Huey, 2007). Some have argued that their occupational environments—spaces of urban impoverishment, high crime and few resources—have necessitated that frontline officers take on a social work role, serving to fill in gaps in the social safety net to prevent further harm to vulnerable people (Wallace, 1965; Blumberg et al., 1973). Waddington (1993), for example, points to the unique resources and institutional connections upon which police can draw in order to secure assistance for those in need. We might also note public reliance on 9-1-1 and the fact that the police remain one of the few 24/7 service providers who can be mobilized to deal with various situations (Skogan, 1999).

In short, to once again echo Bittner (1990), there are few problems in which the police have not been involved in one way or another. This, by consequence, means that there are many avenues through which PMI can become 'police property'. It is these situations under the crime, disorder, and public safety umbrellas that we dive into herein.

The Disordered and the Disorderly

Before we proceed with outlining the data drawn upon for this book, as well as the outline of the book itself, it is necessary to briefly discuss how the police come to the determination that an individual with whom they are interacting may have a mental illness. It has been well-documented in the research literature that officers rely heavily on behavioural cues to assess a situation—such as visual and/or auditory hallucinations or other erratic behaviour (Bittner, 1967; Bohrman et al., 2018; McTackett & Thomas, 2017). Furthermore, officers also rely upon other sources of information, such as prior contact history (McTackett & Thomas, 2017), dispatch communications, and/or bystanders, friends, family, or neighbours (Bohrman et al., 2018). Historically, the information noted above was all that was available, and therefore was what police had to rely upon to make on-the-spot assessments. While these sources are undoubtedly helpful in many cases to inform officers as to whether an individual may have a mental illness, work by Bohrman et al. (2018)—the only empirical attempt to explicitly examine how police assess for mental illness—suggests there may be limitations to many of these information sources. For instance, when it comes to dispatch information, the dispatchers themselves may have not been informed as to whether an individual may have a mental illness thus leaving the responding officer(s) to come to this determination on their own when they arrive on scene. Furthermore, information from bystanders, friends, family, and/or neighbours could similarly be incomplete or even inaccurate or misleading. As such, when faced with these limitations, Bohrman et al. (2018) report that officers tend to rely on their own observations to determine as to whether an individual may have a mental illness.

Officer observations, however, are themselves open to limitations. As officers interviewed by Bohrman et al. (2018) note, and as other studies have similarly observed (Kesic & Thomas, 2014; McTackett & Thomas, 2017), officers are at times unable to distinguish between signs of mental illness and symptoms associated with substance use. Although the prevalence of such situations is not currently known, it is plausible to assume that there are likely instances in which officers mistook the former as the latter and thus opted for a particular course of action under the pretence that the individual was intoxicated as opposed to action that would have been more appropriate given the *true* circumstances of the interaction, such as transport to the local hospital or psychiatric facility.

Perhaps not surprisingly, given the prevalence of mental health-related calls police attend, and the inadequate nature of some of the information upon which they were historically forced to rely in order to make determinations, Canadian police services are increasingly turning to technological solutions. Although not in use during the time in which our data was collected, today, several Canadian police services are relying on a mobile mental health application (or 'app') for assisting officers with clinical decision-making in the field. The app is a mental health screener developed by a consortium of mental health professionals for use by first responders (Hirdes et al., 2019; Hoffman et al., 2016), known as the interRAI Brief

Mental Health Screener. The screener consists of a series of questions intended to assist police with determining if they are dealing with someone with a mental health issue, who may need emergency psychiatric treatment. Information entered by officers, and the results, can then be electronically transmitted to personnel at the nearest emergency facility.

The Data

To explore the different ways in which mental health has become 'police property', we draw on the results of two separate ethnographies of police practices in Canada. The first study combined systematic social observation with interviews and analysis of calls for service data to examine policing of antisocial behaviour. From this study, we draw on two data sources: field notes supplemented with data from in-depth qualitative interviews conducted with 16 participants. Field notes captured events that occurred during 74 police ride-alongs, which comprised approximately 637 h of observations. In total, 406 police-citizen encounters were documented. The second study similarly drew on systematic social observation from 74 ride-alongs to investigate police decision-making by frontline officers. The resulting sample included 402 police-citizen encounters. Of these, 67 involved situations in which an individual was dealing with mental health issues and/or mental illness was the main or a contributing factor.

How do we know if a civilian involved in a police encounter had a mental health condition? We relied on three sources. The first was information from police data provided to the researcher by the officer with whom she was riding. Police record management systems (RMS) typically allow for individuals with a history of police involvement to be 'flagged' for different conditions, including 'M' for *Mental Health* or *Mental Instability*. For example, a male in one encounter is described as 'Flag M'. The second method of identifying a possible mental health issue was through direct references to an individual's mental health and/or relevant diagnoses offered through interactions with officers by the individual him, her, or themselves, or by friends and family members, psychiatric or social workers. From the field notes in encounter 261: 'The complainant (#345) advises she is a schizophrenic and feels like she is being threatened'. Third, for each citizen encounter, the researcher filled out encounter sheets that included her observations, including her feeling that an individual may have been dealing with a mental illness. These sheets were not only reviewed by the attending officer but were also actively discussed. In situations where there was agreement between the researcher and the officer as to a potential mental health condition, the data was included in this study. In those instances where there was not common agreement, the data was excluded. To illustrate: one such case involved a 24-year-old male who had been flagged for a previous suicide attempt but for whom there was no mental health flag in the police Records Management System (RMS). The call involved a burning vehicle (a GMC Jimmy) which the young man had been driving. From the field notes: 'His demeanour was bizarre given the situation. He didn't seem shook up about anything. It was like he didn't have a care in the world. Periodically commenting and laughing about what the officer seems to care about'. Whereas the researcher found the behaviour strange and potentially indicative of a mental health issue, the officer offered a different interpretation: '[The man] doesn't own the Jimmy, have an emotional contact, or vested interest' (field notes).

To help provide some context, we present some basic information on: (1) How the call was originally dispatched; (2) Who initiated the call; and (3) The known demographic characteristics of the PMI involved in the call for service.

In the current public discourse on police reform, particularly in relation to mental health calls, various arguments have been put forward to the effect that police should no longer be involved in responding to calls involving PMI. The reality is, as the Paquet-Korchinski case among others illustrate, in many instances police may be unaware of the underlying dynamics of a call. For example, an incident reported as a physical assault of a family member could involve many unknown variables, from intoxication to a victim with Asperger's syndrome, to mental health issues or ongoing domestic violence. As we document through analysis of our data in subsequent chapters, as police arrive onsite and gain more information, is when they often become aware they are dealing with an actual or potential mental-health related cal (see Table 1.1)

Table 1.1 Initial dispatched call codes

Call type	Total
Check well-being	13
Attempted suicide	8
Domestic dispute (other)	7
Mentally ill person	5
Unwanted contact	3
Domestic dispute	3
Person stop	3
Theft under $5000	2
Assault	2
Follow-up	2
Disturbance	2
Threatening	1
Offensive weapon	1
Missing person	1
Child custody and access	1
Fire (arson)	1
Dispute	1
Intoxicated person	1
Unwanted person (trespass)	1
Dangerous condition	1
Suspicious person	1

(continued)

Table 1.1 (continued)

Call type	Total
Driving complaint	1
Animal complaint	1
By-law complaint	1
Vehicle stop	1
Administrative notice (911)	1
By-law complaint	1
Other (no recorded dispatch code)	1
Total	67

Another caveat that needs to be considered when relying on initial dispatch codes to understand police calls for service is that, as more information becomes available to officers on scene about people and events, the call type code can be changed. In 16 cases (or approximately 24% of calls observed), the call type was recoded by officers immediately following the event. In three instances ($n = 3$) the code type was changed to 'Mentally Ill Person'. Other call types entered during recoding included: 'Check Well-being' ($n = 3$), 'Arrest' ($n = 3$), 'Sudden Death' ($n = 1$), 'Domestic Dispute (other)' ($n = 1$), 'Threatening' ($n = 1$), 'Drugs' ($n = 1$), 'Missing person' ($n = 1$), 'Personal fraud (identity)' ($n = 1$), and 'Dispute' ($n = 1$).

As a result of media reports of police interactions with PMI that tend to focus on the more sensationalized cases involving fatalities or other negative outcomes, there is a not uncommon misconception in public discourse that police come into contact with PMI through either self-initiated proactive policing or as a result of a criminal event involving family members, businesses, or members of the public. We located several examples of such reporting, featuring headlines like 'He Went Crazy and Started Stabbing People': Vancouver Police Corner and Kill Man on Wild Stabbing Spree' (PostMedia News, 2015) and 'Erratic, Sword-Wielding Man Arrested in Downtown Kelowna' (Rodriguez, 2021). In our sample, as can be seen in Table 1.1, the majority of calls were significantly more mundane and less violent than these headlines might suggest. They were also more frequently initiated by family members or the PMI him/her/themselves as we document in Table 1.2:

One of the problems we faced was collecting demographic data. Where possible, information regarding gender, age, and race/ethnicity was recorded in field notes. This information was gleaned either through verbal interactions witnessed between officers and individuals on scene or through attributes ascribed through researcher observation. We acknowledge there are significant limitations with relying on the latter, particularly when it comes to attributions of race/ethnicity. We will discuss this limitation in more detail shortly.

The gender breakdown of our sample included 23 women ($n = 23$), 45 men ($n = 45$), and 1 unknown gender ($n = 1$). As some readers might have immediately noticed, our total number of PMI in this sample is 69 ($n = 69$), which is two greater

Table 1.2 Identity of the individual who initiated the call

Call initiator	Total
Family member	18
PMI him/her/themself	16
General public	6
Police-initiated	6
Social worker	5
Retail business	5
Neighbour	4
Psychiatric facility	3
Transit	1
School	1
Unknown	2
Total	67

Table 1.3 Known age of the PMI

Age group	Total
12–17[a]	8
18–302	19
31–45	15
46–60	12
60+	3
Age unknown	12
Total	69

[a]In the province in which these studies were conducted, the legal age of adulthood is 18. Anyone under 18 is considered a minor

than the number of events we recorded. Simply put, this is because two incidents involved more than one individual with a mental illness. For example, during an investigation of a transit dispute, police officers discovered that two of the individuals had been flagged as 'M' for mental health issues in their RMS, which shaped how they opted to respond to the situation (with a verbal warning).

When it was possible to record an individual's age, this was done. Unfortunately, this was not always the case, and we recorded a relatively high number of unknowns, which we acknowledge as another limitation. That said, we present the known ages in Table 1.3.

As we have extensively documented elsewhere (see Huey et al., 2021), one of the greatest challenges facing would be police reformers in Canada, and to varying extents in other countries, is the problematic nature of collecting race- and ethnicity-based data. Many of the arguments advanced for the need for systematic reform centre on racial and economic disparities in the criminal justice system. This has been no less the case when it comes to arguing for the removal or reduction of police involvement with PMI. Numerous articles, commentaries, and other forms of public opinion following the death of Ms. Korchinski-Paquet and other high profile police fatalities of Black and/or Indigenous people have prompted some within activist communities to claim that 'being Black, Indigenous and/or living with mental health conditions is criminalized' and therefore policy-makers should 'end police response to mental health and wellness related calls, including substance use, domestic abuse, and mental health emergencies' (Seon, 2020).

The unfortunate reality is there are significant problems with the use of any race-based criminal justice data. In policing, such data has historically relied on officer observation and subsequent attribution of a racial or ethnic identity. Anyone familiar with research into the frequency of errors that can be made in such attributions can see why this practice would be highly problematic (see, for example, a meta-analytic review by Meissner & Brigham, 2001). Perhaps not surprisingly, many Canadian police services attempted to side-step the issue several decades ago by imposing an 'informal ban' of sorts on the collection of race-based data (Wortley, 1999). Today, such data is routinely collected within police RMS; however, being mindful of the inaccuracies of such data, Statistics Canada has not previously attempted to collect it as part of the national Uniform Crime Reporting (UCR) data. We understand this is set to change, and that race and ethnicity-based data will be included in the UCR in the future, although how such information will be standardized remains unclear (Tunney, 2020).

All of the above is intended to highlight the ongoing problems with trying to capture, use, and draw assumptions and inferences based on the race/ethnicity of PMI. In the studies we document here, we too chose to side-step attempts at collecting race-based information unless this information was shared by the PMI at some point during the encounter. Thus, our sample of 67 encounters involving 69 PMI includes one Black individual ($n = 1$), one Hispanic individual ($n = 1$), and one Indigenous individual ($n = 1$).

The Book

Drawing on this unique data and the relevant policing literature, we provide a detailed examination of two aspects of the police role and mandate that bring police officers into contact with PMI: *public safety, crime response,* and *keeping the peace*.

In Chap. 2 we explore the *public safety* dimensions of the police role. In particular, we draw on the data collected to examine six ways in which police interact with PMI: (1) conducting apprehensions under provincial and territorial mental health legislation; (2) investigating reports of PMI who have been reported missing from home, shelters, or from hospitals or in-patient facilities; (3) conducting wellness checks on individuals who may be at risk of harm; (4) responding to threats of suicide, (5) follow-up calls; and (6) calls for other matters which only reveal to include PMI upon responding to the scene.

The focus of Chap. 3 is *crime response*, which occurs when police are mobilized or initiate responses to situations involving actual or potential crime and disorder. The interactions we examine include police interactions with PMI who are victims of crime and/or suspects in crime and/or disorder calls. And, recognizing that much of what police actually do entails simply trying to avert potential problems, we also look at how PMI can variously become the subjects of disorder complaints and possible crime calls (as potential victims and/or suspects).

Utilizing both interview data and researcher field observations, in Chap. 4 we also explore police perceptions of the roles they play in the lives of those with mental illness and, in turn, how the demands for police to respond to situations involving mental illness—to 'do something!'—place demands on police that can shape how they view and interact with PMI.

Much of the recent public discourse on contemporary policing has focused on diverting mental health-related calls for service, as well as funding, away from police in order to adopt more holistic, 'upstream' approaches. In the final chapter of this book, we shift the focus away from the present towards envisioning possibilities for the future. To do so, we draw on insights gleaned from the data presented throughout this book to offer both immediate and mid-term practical solutions for reducing the 'footprint' of policing in the lives of individuals with mental illness.

References

Baum, D. (1997). *Smoke and mirrors: The war on drugs and the politics of failure*. Back Bay Books.
Bayley, D. H. (1994). *Police for the future*. Oxford University Press.
Benson, B. L., Rausmussen, D. W., & Sollars, D. L. (1995). Police bureaucracies, their incentives, and the war on drugs. *Public Choice, 83*, 21–45.
Bittner, E. (1967). The police on skid-row: A study of peace keeping. *American Sociological Review, 32*(5), 699–715.
Bittner, E. (1990). *Aspects of police work*. Northeastern University Press.
Blumberg, L., Shipley, T. E., Jr., & Shandler, I. W. (1973). *Skid row and its alternatives: Research and recommendations from Philadelphia*. Temple Univ. Press.
Bohrman, C., Wilson, A., Watson, A., & Draine, J. (2018). How police officers assess for mental illnesses. *Victims & Offenders, 13*(8), 1077–1092.
Charette, Y., Crocker, A. G., & Billette, I. (2011). The judicious judicial dispositions juggle: Characteristics of police interventions involving people with a mental illness. *Canadian Journal of Psychiatry, 56*(11), 677–685. https://doi.org/10.1177/070674371105601106
Coleman, T., & Cotton, D. (2010). Reducing risk and improving outcomes of police interactions with people with mental illness. *Journal of Police Crisis and Negotiation, 10*(1–2), 39–57.
Cooper, H. L. F. (2015). War on drugs policing and police brutality. *Substance Use and Misuse, 50*(8–9), 1188–1194.
Cray, E. (1972). *The enemy in the streets: Police malpractice in America*. Anchor Books.
D.A.R.E. (2021). *The history of D.A.R.E.* https://dare.org/history/
Deener, A., Erie, S., Kogan, V., & Stuart, F. (2013). *Planning Los Angeles: The changing politics of neighborhood and downtown development* (pp. 385–412). The Uncertain Future.
Emsley, C. (2003). The birth and development of the police. In T. Newburn (Ed.), *Handbook of policing* (pp. 66–83). Willan Publishing.

Hirdes, J., van Everdingen, C., Ferris, J., Franco-Martin, M., Fries, B., et al. (2019). The inter RAI suite of mental health assessment instruments: An integrated system for the continuum of care. *Frontiers in Psychiatry, 10*, 926–956.

Hoffman, R., Hirdes, J., Brown, G., Dubin, J., & Barbaree, H. (2016). The use of a brief mental health screener to enhance the ability of police officers to identify persons with serious mental disorders. *International Journal of Law and Psychiatry, 47*(1), 28–35.

Huey, L. (2007). *Negotiating demands: The politics of skid row policing in Edinburgh, San Francisco, and Vancouver*. University of Toronto Press.

Huey, L., Ferguson, L., & Vaughan, A. D. (2021). The limits of our knowledge: Tracking the size and scope of police involvement with persons with mental illness. *Facets: Journal of the Royal Society of Canada*. https://www.facetsjournal.com/doi/full/10.1139/facets-2021-0005?utm_content=bufferd07ea&utm_medium=social&utm_source=twitter.com&utm_campaign=buffer&

Kesic, D., & Thomas, S. D. (2014). Do prior histories of violence and mental disorders impact on violent behaviour during encounters with police? *International Journal of Law and Psychiatry, 37*(4), 409–414.

Lamb, H., Weinberger, L., & DeCuir, W. (2002). The police and mental health. *Psychiatric Services, 53*(10), 1266–1271.

Lee, J. A. (1981). Some structural aspects of police deviance in relations with minority groups. In C. Shearing (Ed.), *Organisational police deviance*. Butterworth.

Lynch, M. (2012). Theorizing the role of the 'war on drugs' in US punishment. *Theoretical Criminology, 16*(2), 175–199.

McDaniel, J. (2019). Reconciling mental health, public policing and police accountability. *The Police Journal, 92*(1), 72–94.

McSheehy, W. (1979). *Skid row*. G.K. Hall & Co.

McTackett, L. J., & Thomas, S. D. M. (2017). Police perceptions of irrational unstable behaviours and use of force. *Journal of Police and Criminal Psychology, 32*(2), 163–171. https://doi.org/10.1007/s11896-016-9212-y

Meissner, C., & Brigham, J. (2001). Thirty years of investigating the own-race bias in memory for faces: A meta-analytic review. *Psychology, Public Policy and Law, 7*(1), 3–35.

Philips, D. (1977). *Crime and authority in Victorian England*. Croom Helm.

PostMedia News (2015). 'He went crazy and started stabbing people': Vancouver police corner and kill man on wild stabbing spree. *National Post*. Available at: https://nationalpost.com/news/canada/he-went-crazy-and-startedstabbing-people-vancouver-police-corner-and-kill-man-on-wild-stabbing-spree.

Reiner, R. (1992). *The politics of the police*. Harvester Wheatsheaf.

Rodriguez, M. (2021). Erratic, sword-wielding man arrested in downtown Kelowna. *Vernon Morning Star*. Available at: https://www.vernonmorningstar.com/news/erratic-sword-wielding-man-arrested-in-downtown-kelowna/.

Rogers, A. (1990). Policing mental disorder: Controversies, myths and realities. *Social Policy and Administration, 24*(2), 226–236.

Rosenbaum, D. P. (2007). Just say no to D.A.R.E. *Criminology and Public Policy, 6*, 815–824.

Sellers, C., Sullivan, C., Veysey, B., & Shane, J. (2005). Responding to persons with mental illnesses: Police perspectives on specialized and traditional practices. *Behavioual Science and the Law, 23*(5), 647–657.

Seon, Q. (2020). Black, indigenous, and people of colour are criminalized and killed for their mental health conditions. *The McGill Daily*. https://www.mcgilldaily.com/2020/07/policing-mental-health-and-wellness/#close-modal

Sherman, L. W. (2013). The rise of evidence-based policing: Targeting, testing, and tracking. *Crime and Justice, 42*(1), 377–451.

Shore, K., & Lavoie, J. (2019). Exploring mental health-related calls for police service: A Canadian study of police officers as 'frontline mental health workers'. *Policing: A Journal of Policy and Practice, 13*(2), 157–171.

References

Skogan, W. (1999). *Community policing: Chicago style*. Oxford University Press.

Skogan, W., & Frydl, K. (2004). Fairness and effectiveness in policing: The evidence. In *Fairness and effectiveness in policing*. The National Academies Press.

Stuart, F. (2016). *Down, out, and under arrest: Policing and everyday life in skid row*. University of Chicago Press.

Teplin, L., & Pruett, N. (1992). Police as streetcorner psychiatrist: Managing the mentally ill. *International Journal of Law and Psychiatry, 15*(2), 139–156.

Tribolet-Hardy, F., Kesic, D., & Thomas, S. (2015). Police management of mental health crisis situations in the community: Status quo, current gaps and future directions. *Policing and Society, 25*(3), 294–307.

Tunney, C. (2020). Statistics Canada to start collecting race-based crime data. *CBC Online*. .https://www.cbc.ca/news/politics/statistics-canada-race-data-police-1.5650273

Waddington, P. A. J. (1993). *Calling the police interpretation of, and response to, calls for assistance from the police*. Avebury.

Wallace, S. E. (1965). *Skid row as a way of life*. Bedminster Press.

Weisburd, D., & Braga, A. A. (2006). Introduction: Understanding police innovation. In D. Weisburd & A. A. Braga (Eds.), *Police innovation: Contrasting perspectives* (1st ed., pp. 1–23). Cambridge University Press.

West, S. L., & O'Neal, K. K. (2004). Project D.A.R.E. outcome effectiveness revisited. *American Journal of Public Health, 94*(6), 1027–1029.

Wilson, J. Q., & Kelling, G. (1982). Broken windows. *Atlantic Monthly, 249*, 29–38.

Wilson, J. Q. (1968). *Varieties of police behavior*. Harvard University Press.

Wiseman, J. P. (1970). *Stations of the lost: The treatment of skid row alcoholics*. Prentice Hall.

Wood, J., Watson, A., & Fulambarker, A. (2017). The "gray zone" of police work during mental health encounters: Findings from an observational study in Chicago. *Police Quarterly, 20*(1), 81–105.

Wortley, S. (1999). A Northern taboo: Research on race, crime, and criminal justice in Canada. *Canadian Journal of Criminology, 41*(2), 261–274.

Chapter 2
The Public Safety Role

Not all police interactions with PMI will involve criminal matters. Police are also frequently called upon to deal with citizens in situations in which someone's health or safety may be at risk. Under the umbrella of 'public safety', we examine six ways in which police interact with PMI in non-criminal circumstances. The first are 'mental health apprehensions'—that is, cases where police officers take someone into custody for the purposes of escorting them to the nearest designated hospital or psychiatric facility for intake and treatment. As we describe, in some instances police must make 'on the spot' assessments of whether someone meets the threshold criteria for apprehension; in other cases, police are directed to apprehend as a result of a provincial committal notice. The second type of interaction we examine is missing persons calls, wherein a citizen has intentionally left home or absconded from a treatment or other facility. The third call type is the 'wellness' check, during which officers are mobilized to verify the health and well-being of someone who is deemed by a complainant as being 'at risk' or in some type of peril. The fourth call type involves the most serious of these cases: those involving threats of suicide. Fifth, we briefly touch upon follow-up calls, which are proactive visits to check on the well-being of vulnerable individuals, before concluding with an example of calls that do not or would not initially strike one as involving PMI. As we detail, when individuals are in crisis, they, or friends or family, may mobilize police to prevent harm. Finally, we will also touch upon calls for other matters in which it is not immediately clear that the call involves someone with a mental illness.

Mental Health Apprehensions

Provincial and territorial mental health legislation creates a mandated role for police to apprehend PMI who are under a warrant or other authorization ordering an individual to be apprehended and transported for psychological examination and treatment. The *Mental Health Act* in several Canadian jurisdictions stipulate that the police may be called upon to bring someone to a facility for a psychological assessment, either by application from a physician or an order from a justice of the peace. These are typically situations in which someone is already under some form of in-patient or community treatment order, but who has not complied with treatment demands. When that happens, mental health professionals call upon police to respond. One such example can be found in Encounter 101. When a male patient left a psychiatric ward, hospital staff issued a 'Form 9' for him, which directs the police to apprehend and return him to their custody for medical treatment. He was subsequently located by officers on his girlfriend's porch and returned. It is this function that has caused some researchers to liken the police role in mental health calls to that of a 'swift, free taxi-service' (Andoh, 1998, p. 350).

The *Mental Health Act* can also be invoked to apprehend and transport to hospital for assessment an individual who has, or is threatening to, cause bodily harm against themselves or another person. Such a situation can, for example, stem from a call for help from family members, who may lack the knowledge or resources to deal with an individual in a state of crisis. As Jennifer Wood et al. (2017, p. 88) have observed, such crises can 'emerge from a lack of medication adherence and a family's inability to handle a situation'. An example of this type of situation can be found in the details of Encounter 367. Police were dispatched to a 'domestic dispute' between a father and adult son by the mother, who was described as 'very upset and hard to understand'. As the officer who takes the call is relatively junior, two units and a Sergeant also attend. Once there, more information emerges. Both males are intoxicated and have been engaged in a verbal argument. The son, who has been diagnosed with depression and anxiety, has not been taking his medication. According to the mother, his prescription for anti-depressants has not been filled because no one knows what has happened to his prescription. He is now emotionally distressed and suicidal, repeatedly yelling, 'I don't give a fuck anymore'. Officers on scene learn he is upset because 'his father told him he is going to go buy a gun and bullets tomorrow and give it to him so he can kill himself' (field notes).

Police are all too keenly aware of the limitations they face in crafting a perfect solution (Bittner, 1990; Schulenberg, 2016). Leaving this male at home while emotions are running high, and he is potentially suicidal, is clearly not desirable. However, in taking him to a hospital under the *Mental Health Act*, they run the risk that the psychiatrist may not agree this individual meets the necessary threshold for admission—a problem for which police officers have long had to devise compromise solutions to avoid a future 'problem' (Bittner, 1990). If released, a potentially suicidal male could be forced by circumstance to return to a volatile situation at home. The officers conduct some contingency planning and then proceed to explain their solution: they will execute a *Mental Health Act* apprehension, as well as laying a charge against the young male for Breach of the Peace. The rationale for the latter is seen as 'a type of insurance policy': if he is not detained at the hospital, they can use the outstanding charge to place him in lockup over night until 'until everyone calms down' (field notes). That police should rely on this strategy as a backup plan is of little surprise: separating feuding parties is a standard peacekeeping tactic (Bittner, 1967; Brown, 1988).

Another case similarly illustrates how calls dispatched for ostensibly one cause can quickly become encounters leading to a mental health apprehension. Encounter 280 began as an 'unwanted contact' call when an individual called 9-1-1 to report someone stalking him in a grocery parking lot. In this case, the complainant was known to officers, as he had called with a similar story the day before. After listening to his concerns over being stalked,

> The officers began talking to the complainant and telling him that they do not have sufficient grounds to lay any charges for harassment, assault, or stalking. The officers then began to ask where the individual previously resided. The man stated that he lived in [city name removed], but he moved because the police did not do anything when people gave him a hard time. The officers asked the man if he had a mental illness because his behaviour was 'too paranoid'. The man said no.

Given both his current behaviour and previous history with police, the officers disagree. They see themselves as having sufficient grounds to apprehend him under the provincial *Mental Health Act*. In this instance, the admitting psychiatrist also agrees, as the complainant is involuntarily admitted.

Another encounter is initially dispatched as a 'missing person' call; however, the individual is not missing, but rather has absconded from hospital property and hospital staff want her returned. She is not, in any sense, 'missing'. Both the hospital and police not only know her location—she is on a local transit bus—but she is accompanied by two hospital security officers. The issue is the security personnel lack the legal authority to force her return, so police are mobilized instead. When officers arrived, they find a bus driving away and an upset woman with two security guards in tow. While they work to calm her, the hospital prepares the appropriate paperwork to allow an officer to apprehend her and bring her back to the hospital.

In theory, one might expect that once the decision to admit someone for psychiatric treatment, the police role would be over. However, as with the *Mental Health Act* process more generally, mental health facilities often rely on police powers of coercion to ensure patient compliance—framed in the language of 'safety'—rather than utilizing hospital security or other means (Wood et al., 2021). Fieldnotes from Encounter 280 describe what happened once the complainant was told he was being admitted for a psychiatric evaluation:

> [He] was not pleased by this and said that he was going to leave, or else he is going to 'sue the fucking police and the fucking hospital'. The hospital staff then left and the two officers entered the room. The second officer explained to [him] that his patience was running thin and that they can either accompany him to the psych ward, or they will physically take him to the psych ward. [The man] complied and was handcuffed behind his back.
>
> When we arrived to the psych ward, one of the nurses directed us to a room where there were two beds, a washroom, and a closet to hang your clothes. The officers gave the nurses the album that [he] brought with him. [The man] stated that he needed that album otherwise he was going to cause trouble. He began swearing, so the officers placed him back into handcuffs and the nurse told the officers to accompany him to a room on the other side of the ward. This new room only had 1 bed and was a lockable room only accessible with a key fob. The officers removed the man's handcuffs, placed him in the room, and the nurse locked the door.

The stated rationale for police involvement in moving patients under such circumstances is 'safety'; however, there is a longstanding belief among officers that this is a form of 'dirty work' which they are called upon to undertake, so that hospital staff need not resort to physical violence or other forms of coercion (Bittner, 1990).

Missing Persons

As we saw with the case of the woman who was reported as 'missing' after having absconded from a psychiatric facility, in some instances hospitals and other facilities are aware of the fact an individual has left their premises and mobilize police in response. In other situations, however, staff remain unaware that someone has 'gone missing' until they are notified that an individual has been 'found'—usually through unrelated reports from businesses or members of the public. One such example involved an individual who was technically missing twice within the space of one call. Police were first dispatched to attend a minor disturbance call. The employee of a local donut shop had called to complain about an individual, who had asked the employee for a ride back to the hospital before soliciting money from customers to purchase a soft drink. When police arrived 10 min later, the man has disappeared. However, based on his comments to the employee, they contact the local psychiatric facility, which discover he is 'missing'. From that call, police were able to learn an identity and a description. They also learned he was a routine absconder with diabetes, who leaves the hospital to find ways to acquire sugary treats. Of particular concern: 'If he has high sugar levels, he will douse himself in water and be soaking wet' (field notes). As the temperature is then -14 °C, the Sergeant on scene realizes the absconding patient is in potential danger and switches the call type from 'disturbance' to 'missing persons' and puts out a call for other units. As units clear existing calls, they are dispatched to this one, and the airwaves are cleared of all non-emergency calls. Officers have already canvassed nearby businesses, so a larger ground search is ordered. Over time, 19 units join the call, including one Sergeant, 11 patrol vehicles, three emergency response, two detective and two K9 units. One of these units is assigned to the hospital to receive more information and to be present if the person returns. Notifications are issued to local transit companies, hospitals, restaurants, and convenience stores. Several hours later, an unknown person is seen wandering the grounds of the hospital and the missing person is identified. By this point, he has wandered over some eight miles in sub-zero temperatures. The field notes raise an important question:

> Why didn't [the] Hospital report him missing? Is it because he called a few times? If he is a Form 4 involuntary in-patient and he has done this many times before…why is he issued a two hour pass in the first place?

Police are also mobilized to attend missing calls by worried family members. Encounter 106 involves a 21-year-old woman with substance use disorder. She is also a victim-witness in a domestic violence case, which places her at some potential risk, raising concern for her well-being. So too does the fact that the last time she was in police custody she attempted suicide. Two units and an Acting Sergeant attend her residence, discover her home unlocked and begin searching her apartment. Aware of her history of mental health issues, the officers then make calls to mental health facilities, local hospitals and to the neighbouring police service to track down her boyfriend (the accused in the domestic violence case). Several hours later, during a police follow-up, the victim-witness answers the door. She is completely uninterested in why the police are there, and slightly hostile. From the field notes:

> The officers explain the reason for their visit which is to clear her father's missing person's report he filed earlier in the day. As she is a valuable witness for the pending assault case and the missing persons report there was a serious concern for her safety and well-being. Her response is, "Can I go now?"

Wellness Checks

Wellness checks, also known as 'well-being checks' or 'compassionate to locate' calls, are calls for service in which police are asked to verify the safety and well-being of an individual for whom there is concern. Concerns might involve possible accidents, threats over harm to self or others, or incapacitation due to illness. With this type of call, we have not only field data, but also direct experience. One of the authors received a wellness check once, when her husband had been unable to reach her by phone when he was out of town. Knowing she was planning on painting that day using a ladder, he feared she had an accident and called the New York State Police, who then called the local police department. Later that night, a uniformed officer arrived on her doorstep and proceeded to ask a series of questions about her mental health and whether she had intentions to harm herself. Such questions are not unusual in these types of situations, as wellness checks frequently have a mental health component.

As the personal example above illustrates, family members are a frequent source of calls requesting wellness checks. One desperate father had called in a missing person report and, based on concerns by the father that the young man has bipolar disorder, a history of suicide attempts, and is presently 'very unstable', the attending officer broadcasts a 'compassionate to locate' to all divisions. Another encounter similarly entails responding to a distressed mother dealing with a 14-year-old girl with a history of self-injurious behaviour ('cutting') and running away.

In media reporting of police encounters with PMI, the typical scenario involves a bystander or concerned family member dialling 9-1-1. What is perhaps less well known is that in many instances police are dispatched by the individual themselves during periods of extreme emotional and/or mental crisis. Encounter 138 begins with a 27-year-old male, who dials 9-1-1 from the parking lot of a local fire hall. Upon arrival, the officer finds someone who is emotionally distraught, unkempt, and threating to harm himself or others. He explains to the officer, that his mother is going through a romantic breakup and is devastated. He is angry and disturbed over seeing her 'in so much pain and crying all the time' that he 'wants to hurt someone to get rid of the feeling inside' (field notes). Recognizing this as an extreme reaction, the officer brings him for psychiatric observation on a voluntary apprehension.

Another example of a self-initiated wellness check entails a call from an emotionally distraught male with a lengthy criminal history, who is dealing with depression. He is currently on bail and is asking officers to arrest him because he wants to 'go to jail and get it over with'. He claims to be drunk, and thus in violation of his bail conditions, and is demanding to be taken to a local correctional facility. When police advise they cannot simply arrest him, he proposes to be taken to a hospital instead. Given his current condition, and the fact he has 'large, long cuts across his torso of previous self-harm' (field notes), they agree he likely meets the criteria for a mental health apprehension and transport him to the local hospital.

Dropped calls to 9-1-1 by PMI also initiate wellness checks. Encounter 335 illustrates this process: an emotionally distressed male dials 9-1-1 and yells for the Emergency Communications operator to 'send the fucking cops now' before hanging up. When police locate him at his father's home, he is clearly highly upset. He is the complainant in a criminal case involving a purported sexual assault and he states he was in the forest when he called police. While there, he 'saw the people in the forest who sexually assaulted him' (field notes).

Wellness checks are also initiated by mental health agencies and other service and treatment providers out of concern for clients. One such example occurs in Encounter 240. A mental health worker has received a call from a client, who advises he is going to cut off his hands and then try to kill himself. When police arrive, they discover the man has left and taken his car. They then issue a radio broadcast with the wellness check code ('928') and a description of his car to other patrol cars to be on the lookout for this individual.

Suicide

The extent to which mental health has become viewed as 'police property' within and outside of the criminal justice system is no more apparent than in calls initiated by mental health and social work organizations that could, in practical terms, very likely be handled internally without mobilizing police resources. We saw this with missing persons cases, and we see it again in calls involving 'attempt suicide'. One such example was a call from staff at a community organization that offers addiction and other treatment services. They were concerned over an intoxicated client, who had stopped taking his psychotropic drugs, was depressed and had been talking about ending his life. When police arrived, he voluntarily agreed to be brought to a hospital for a mental health assessment and was escorted there by an officer.

In our sample of observed interactions, family and friends were the most frequent initiators of calls involving suicide threats. In both studies, family members mobilized the police in response to text messages or other forms of communication that either hinted at or directly stated an individual was experiencing suicidal ideation. In some situations, loved ones were not nearby and thus requesting police assistance was seen as the fastest and safest solution. In other instances, mobilizing the police offers a faint hope that someone will receive the psychiatric and other resources they desperately require. That police are seen as street-level gatekeepers to mental health resources is a prevalent, if not always accurate belief given the difficulties police themselves admit in securing those resources (as we discuss in further detail in Chap. 4; see also Patch & Arrigo, 1999). Regardless, most complainants are likely unaware of this fact when they pick up the phone. To illustrate, a woman called in to 9-1-1 over text messages she and her aunt had received from a cousin who was intimating she was suicidal. The caller requested police 'accompany her [cousin] so that her cousin gets the help she needs' (field notes). As is often the case with emotional crisis calls, the suicidal young woman had a history of similar crises fuelled by substance abuse and untreated mental health issues and the family was reportedly at their 'wits' end' (field notes). The expectation was that if police were called, they could 'do something'.

Whereas most calls from friends and family are out of concern for the immediate well-being of the individual in crisis, sometimes the proposed method selected also presents significant risks to family members or others. Encounter 71 was initiated by a phone call from the son of a distraught woman, whose husband was in the garage threatening to commit suicide by blowing up the family home. From the field notes:

> He has hooked up a propane tank to a heater fan while shutting himself up in the garage. An incendiary device is found, as well as two knives. The road Sergeant breaches the garage and de-escalates the situation. The road is closed and the neighbours are asked to retreat to their basements until further notice.

Mobilizing the police to provide assistance with what some may see as a 'private matter', or in response to a situation fraught with potential threat to their loved one, can spark disagreements among family members. In relation to the latter, we might attribute reluctance—particularly among members of Black, Indigenous or other historically marginalized groups—to cases in which PMI have been shot and killed by police officers. Certainly, this has been a dominant theme in both public and media discourse (King, 2019; Hauck, 2020; Cooke, 2020). We did not observe such dynamics in the interactions that comprise each study, which is very likely explained by the demographic composition of the communities within which the studies were conducted. That said, we did note cases in which family disagreements over 'calling the cops' to deal with a member in crisis were generated by the belief that mental health issues should be treated as a 'private' issue. Once such dispute was witnessed during Encounter 99. A 16-year-old male with mental health, substance use and anger management issues was reported as having 'tried to take a knife and slit his wrists' in response to learning that his father and step-mother had discovered posts on Facebook intimating he had suicidal thoughts (field notes). After his father confiscated the knife, the young man then began striking himself and had to be restrained. The stepmother then called the police. Among the various family dynamics with which police have to deal when they arrive, they discover 'the father was upset with step-mom for calling the police. He feels that he could handle his son's behaviour and what happened that night without police assistance' (field notes). In reviewing the history of calls to this residence, his feelings are not surprising, because this was not the first time the stepmother has called the police: there was a history of parent-child disturbance calls. In this instance, the stepson was unaware the police had been called, and indicates that he 'would have run away if he had known' (field notes). To try to resolve the situation, the officer on scene engaged in what Bittner (1990) has termed 'psychiatric first aid' by focusing on creating distance between the youth and his stepmom, whose behaviour is seen as exacerbating the situation, while working to calm and provide emotional support to the young man. Eventually, the young man is taken for a psychiatric assessment at the local hospital.

A recurring theme in analysing police encounters with PMI is how dynamic these situations can be, morphing from what appears to be one call type when dispatched to a different issue as events unfold. Such shifts necessitate spontaneous changes in police protocol and procedure. Encounter 249 represents a case in point. It begins as a 'suicide attempt' call with a series of 9-1-1 calls from concerned family members. The individual, who had been the subject of a previous suicide attempt call 2 weeks earlier, had sent a text message to a family friend stating he has taken 'a bunch of pills and gin' for the purpose of ending his life (field notes). He has left his home to 'take a walk' and has not been heard from for a few hours. His last text message states he is lost and does not know where he is. With this information, the police response is to shift gears and begin canvassing for him, treating this case now as a high priority missing person call. He is eventually located on a downtown sidewalk, disoriented but conscious from a fall. He is found with four prescription pill bottles, one of which is empty. Police immediately apprehended under the *Mental Health Act* and he is transported to the hospital by ambulance. An officer is sent to wait with him during the evaluation and intake process.

Another example of the dynamic nature of mental health-related calls was provided by an officer during a ride-along, who related the story of one of his most challenging arrests. The encounter described involved an attempted suicide involving a car. Although we have no details as to who initiated the call, it is likely to have been a member of the public who observed this individual driving erratically. At one point, he attempted to drive into another vehicle at 177 km/hour. When the officer arrived on scene, the man had gotten out of the car and stripped naked. Alone, the officer had to try to effect an arrest of a naked, agitated, and highly resistant male. In one of the few instances in this study in which police were either observed using force or spoke of having to use force with a PMI, the officer described trying to knee the male to no effect. When backup arrived, one officer was bit and another had his thumb dislocated. Finally, it took five officers to be able to handcuff him. He was then transported to the hospital for admission to the psychiatric ward.

The bulk of suicide-related calls are resolved without loss of life. However, this is not always the case. Police officers may be dispatched to stop an attempted suicide or to provide assistance to someone who has attempted, only to discover what is termed a 'sudden death'. Encounter 134 began as Priority 1 call for an attempted suicide that had been phoned in to 9-1-1. The frantic mother of a 27-year-old male had found her son unresponsive in the bathtub and believed he had attempted suicide and required emergency assistance. Police arrived to find a scene with blood and vomit all over the bed, walls, and floors, and a male who was clearly deceased in the bathtub. From the field notes:

The 27-year-old male had a lot of prior 933 [domestic dispute], 935 [intoxicated person], and 937 [mentally ill person] calls. He was also on an incredible amount of prescription medications for depression, anxiety, HIV, and other unknown ailments. He took a large number of supplements as well. Altogether, there were three medium sized evidence bags filled with meds. They were everywhere: on the counters, stove, and floor.

Following an autopsy and toxicology report, the death was ruled accidental.

Encounter 134 also helps us to identify another key role the police are called upon to play in relation to suicide and other sudden death cases: death notifications. As many of us are aware from scenes in television and movies, when someone dies suddenly, police may be sent to deliver the information to family members. This occurred, for example, in Encounter 134 described above, wherein a member of another police service had to be dispatched to tell the young man's father that his son and died, and then bring him to meet his wife at the hospital. As with other situations in which individuals may be experiencing emotional or mental crisis, police officers are provided training for this task at the provincial police college, but observational data from other sudden deaths scenes in this study suggest it is one they take on reluctantly.

Follow-up Calls

As we have seen, most police actions involving PMI are not police-initiated. One category we have not previously discussed are 'follow-up' calls. These are proactive visits conducted in order to ascertain the well-being of high risk, vulnerable individuals. One such example can be found in the case of a male with paranoid schizophrenia who has had 114 prior contacts with police. Police crisis response, mental health workers and housing officials are ready to provide assistance, however, he has not provided consent for treatment and there are insufficient grounds for an apprehension under the *Mental Health Act*. Thus, when he gets up and walks away during a coffee with a police officer, there is nothing further they can do for him.

'Hidden' PMI Calls

Some driving-related complaints—clearly those that do not fall into criminal categories such as impaired driving—represent potential safety issues for which bystanders and others may call 9-1-1 for a police response. Encounter 23 typifies such a call. An anonymous caller indicated that after jumping the curb at the roundabout the vehicle's driver asked for directions, appearing disoriented. The male driver was identified as a 47-year-old male, with a history of substance use, suicidal ideation and mental health issues, for which he was currently on medication.

As we see with Encounter 23, not all encounters involving PMI are the result of calls for service initiated about an individual in obvious crisis. This fact is one of the largely unexamined aspects of arguments to 'defund the police'. Put more succinctly: it is not always apparent when a call is dispatched that it will turn into a mental health call necessitating apprehension or some other response. One such 9-1-1 call began with a motor vehicle collision. The caller reported a vehicle having hit a stop sign in an incident the person described as a 'road rage issue'. What police subsequently found was not only a damaged vehicle with a passenger, but also a 25-year-old male in a state of significant distress:

> The driver is very upset and says his life is completely messed up. He lost his home and is living at the Knights Inn as of yesterday ... [he was] evicted yesterday with only four hours notice to vacate. He then starts talking about killing himself. After the other officer speaks with the driver for 15-20 minutes, sufficient grounds exist for a MHA [*Mental Health Act*] apprehension. The driver has made verbal statements to indicate he is an imminent risk to himself or others (field notes).

At that point, the decision was made to apprehend and transport the individual to the local hospital, as he is clearly seen as a danger to himself and others.

Conclusions

Analysis of data presented in this chapter reveals that a significant portion of police contacts with PMI are for non-crime related calls. Furthermore, the majority of calls observed were initiated by family members, psychiatric facilities, social service providers, businesses, and PMI themselves. Generally speaking, police calls were not proactive—that is, police were mobilized by dispatch as a result of a call for service rather than initiating an activity themselves. One exception to this, briefly noted, is the 'follow-up' call—that is, a visit initiated by police to ascertain the whereabouts and well-being of an individual previously encountered, who is deemed as being at 'high risk' of potential harm or, as we see in the next chapter, of engaging in possible criminal activity. What makes the follow-up call an interesting activity worth further examination is the fact that, despite a wealth of research on police-citizen encounters, to date this type of police action has generated little scholarly attention.

Another aspect of police involvement in mental health-related cases in the public safety realm worth examining is the police role in community death notifications. As we saw in the section on suicide-related calls, officers may be called upon not only to deal with sudden death involving PMI, but they are also tasked with relating this information to family members. The implications of this work, which necessarily entail dealing with emotionally distraught individuals, who may or may not have mental illness themselves, has remained largely unexplored.

References

Andoh, B. (1998). The evolution of the role of the police with special reference to social support and the mental health statutes. *Medicine, Science and the Law, 38*(4), 347–353.

Bittner, E. (1967). The police on skid-row: A study of peace keeping. *American Sociological Review, 32*(5), 699–715.

Bittner, E. (1990). *Aspects of police work*. Northeastern University Press.

Brown, M. (1988). *Working the street: Police discretion and the dilemmas of reform*. Russell Sage.

Cooke, A. (2020). Recent deaths prompt questions about police wellness checks. *CBC News*. https://www.cbc.ca/news/canada/nova-scotia/police-wellness-checks-deaths-indigenous-black-1.5622320

Hauck, G. (2020). Walter Wallace had a mental illness, his family says. Why did police respond? *USA Today*. https://www.usatoday.com/story/news/nation/2020/10/28/walter-wallace-philadelphia-shooting-mental-illness/6053831002/

King, S. (2019). If you are black and in a mental health crisis, 911 can be a death sentence. *The Intercept*. https://theintercept.com/2019/09/29/police-shootings-mental-health/

Patch, P., & Arrigo, B. (1999). Police officer attitudes and use of discretion in situations involving the mentally ill: The need to narrow the focus. *International Journal of Law and Psychiatry, 22*(1), 23–35.

Schulenberg, J. (2016). Police decision-making in the gray zone: The dynamics of police–citizen encounters with mentally ill persons. *Criminal Justice and Behavior, 43*(4), 459–482.

Wood, J., Watson, A., & Barber, C. (2021). What can we expect of police in the face of deficient mental health systems? Qualitative insights from Chicago police officers. *Journal of Psychiatric and Mental Health Nursing, 28*(1), 28–42.

Wood, J., Watson, A., & Fulambarker, A. (2017). The "gray zone" of police work during mental health encounters: Findings from an observational study in Chicago. *Police Quarterly, 20*(1), 81–105.

Chapter 3
Crime Prevention and Response Role

In this chapter, we switch focus to the roles that police play when called upon to respond to PMI as victim or suspect. Although some might think this form of police work would entail a strictly law enforcement orientation, as we show through our analysis, whether an individual is a victim or an alleged offender, responding officers may be required to adopt one of several different potential responses that may have little to do with enforcing the law. Indeed, as has been widely documented (see, for example, Schulenberg, 2016; Shore & Lavoie, 2019), when faced with PMI accused of lesser offenses, officers may exercise discretion, choosing instead to treat the situation as one necessitating a mental health rather than criminal justice response. We document such situations in this chapter and the factors that influence officer decision-making. We also present instances where PMI have been victimized and/or are potential risk of harm, and how police respond to the special needs of this portion of the population.

Although PMI are disproportionately represented among victims of crime (Brink et al., 2011; Frederick et al., 2018), and are also found among those charged with criminal offences (Charette et al., 2014; Schulenberg, 2016), they tend to be uniquely overrepresented among those who become the subjects of disorder complaints (Huey, 2007; Kouyoumdjian et al., 2019). In this chapter, we explore police interactions with PMI who are the subject of such complaints, as well as interactions in which PMI are suspects or potential suspects in criminal cases.

Victim-Complainants

Victimization Calls

Despite the fact PMI are among the most heavily victimized social groups (Teplin et al., 2005), little is known about their rates of reporting. One small-scale Canadian study of 60 PMI explored their perceptions of police interactions, finding that approximately 34% of their sample had had contact with police as a result of criminal victimization (Livingston et al., 2014). Indeed, in the previous chapter, we saw such an example in the case involving a woman who was believed to be at increased risk because she was the victim of domestic violence in a case where she was to testify against her ex-partner.

Encounter 93 is unusual in that it is initiated by a high school guidance counsellor in response to a report by a student that another student has been assaulted. The alleged suspect is the victim's boyfriend, who is said to have slapped her in the face during a dispute. The victim is reluctant to discuss the event, but the details that emerge indicate the boyfriend had confronted her over her use of alcohol as a coping strategy for dealing with anxiety and panic attacks. In apprising the victim's parents as the rough details of the case, it becomes apparent that had the counsellor not called the police, it is unlikely the crime would have been reported. The victim is unwilling to implicate her boyfriend and the parents seem skeptical of their daughter. From the fieldnotes:

> The father minimized anxiety and panic attacks and felt it is drama and attention seeking behaviour. He said this right in front of his daughter. She stared at the floor. My officer advised all parties on the seriousness of domestic violence and why there is little discretion used in respect to laying charges. It is the duty of the police to prevent a reoccurrence. He stated that if her ex-boyfriend is going to be charged there will be no contact conditions attached to his release. When the officer was reviewing these next steps, including court and the resources available to [the victim], the father said, 'we'll just have to see how this plays out.' It almost seems like he doesn't believe her.

Whereas there has been some research to suggest that some PMI do not come forward with allegations of victimization for fear of not being believed by police (Burczyka, 2018), less is known of the role that families and friends can play in discounting the experiences of PMI or dissuading individuals from reporting (Huey & Broll, 2018). Given high rates of victimization within this section of the population, and the possible role that untreated trauma can play in worsening of psychiatric conditions, understanding structural and other barriers to help-seeking behaviour—whether that is through police reporting or not—remains a critical task for researchers.

Another type of police encounter that has similarly drawn little research attention involves calls for service by PMI victims and/or complainants that were subsequently cleared by police as 'unfounded'. Encounter 114 is one such example. It began with a report of 'unwanted contact'. The complainant is a 46-year-old woman, who advises dispatch she had received text messages from her ex-boyfriend. She also states, he called that morning to demand to know the location of his daughter and, if he was not told, he would 'kill everyone' (field notes). From the field notes:

Upon arrival it is clear that [the complainant] is quite intoxicated and her story doesn't make sense. The reality is it is all about her daughter's health card which she falsely believes is required to enter detox. She says it is for her daughter who she believes is a 'meth head.' ...

When trying to sort out the complaint she won't let the officer investigate further by speaking with her daughter. She wants her ex-boyfriend to go through the same pain as her daughter. If she had her way, "I'd murder him."

Ultimately, she wants to cause problems for [the ex-boyfriend] because she blames him for her daughter's drug addiction. She doesn't want to discuss the threats, there are no saved text messages of relevance, and the conversation always directs back to the health card and fears for her daughter not going into detox.

She is extremely repetitive, argues with the officer, raises her voice, and doesn't listen to direction or explanations ...

Dealing with an intoxicated person, who is unstable, repeats everything, claims the officer wasn't listening to her, and none of her story made sense – the manner in which this encounter ended I was able to predict and completely understand. [The] officer finally told her that he was leaving as she didn't want the police to assist her in any way.

Another call observed also relates to a family dispute. As the researcher notes, this is the third time she has attended this residence for a domestic dispute during the period of her fieldwork. Before arrival, the attending officer is advised by the Acting Staff-Sergeant 'to make clear to [her] that she can't keep calling us if she's not in danger' (field notes). However, once there, the officer realizes that the warning will not be effective. The reason for the current call is for the same issue as previous ones: the complainant, a 48-year-old woman, wants her adult son arrested and removed from her residence. The officer patiently explains that her son has not broken the law and they cannot arrest him. They will take him to a shelter for the night, but if she does not want him in her home, then she needs to stop letting him in. From the field notes:

She told the officers at the top of her lungs to "Get the fuck out of her house" and [the] officer that he was stupid. "Do I need to write this down for you?" A lot of restraint is exercised because she's clearly mentally ill.

The officer clearly agrees with the researcher's assessment, because he offers to call the services of the Mobile Crisis Unit. Notes from previous interactions with the complainant show that officers have made the same offer before; however, as happens again, she vehemently refuses. In the car after the encounter, the Sergeant with whom the researcher is conducting the ride-along, 'predicts that she will be in a mental health facility a year from now. However, there is no point taking her right now because the [hospital] won't Form 1 her under the *Mental Health Act* yet' (field notes).

Complainant Calls

As with victimization reports, some of the calls for service initiated by PMI as complainants were concluded as 'unfounded'. One such call involved a woman reporting her neighbour's house on fire. When police and fire crews arrive, there is no fire and the house occupants confirm they are well. An officer then visits the home of the complainant and discovers 'a 51-year-old female who suffers from delusions and hallucinations ... she still tries to convince the officer there is a fire'. The complainant also tells police her house is haunted and she hears things, but it is unclear what she expects the officer to do. In another 'unfounded' encounter, a different complainant alleges she is the victim of harassment from a 'witch' who has put a curse on her. The field notes describe this woman as 'repetitive and her story doesn't make a lot of sense'. The officer, who has formed the opinion she is mentally ill, takes the information and then proceeds to track down the alleged harasser. As there is no evidence in support of the allegation, he simply warns the second woman to stay away from the complainant and closes the file.

Yet another example of this phenomenon is documented in an encounter that begins when a woman calls the police to advise she 'feels like she is being threatened at [her shelter]. The staff are not doing anything about it either. She says she needs help and doesn't feel safe there anymore'. When police arrive, the complainant has left the shelter to return a book to the library. When she returns, the story unfolds. She has been diagnosed with schizophrenia and believes her roommate is saying 'bad things' about her to others, although she cannot articulate any actual threats. She is demanding a new room and wants the police to ensure this happens. The decision is then made to transfer her to another facility with available space. The officer then transports her to this new location.

Disturbance complaints regarding noises are another call type generated by PMI. Here too several 'unfounded' encounters were observed. One such encounter began with the complainant calling in a noise complaint over a barking dog in his apartment complex. When officers arrive, there's no noise. Despite the complainant having requested 'no contact' from police, the officers knock on his door to followup. In response to their questioning, the complainant admits he has serious mental health issues and then begins reviewing each of the services with whom he has contact. The officers listen to him patiently for over 30 minutes. While some might view their response as politeness, the researcher observes: 'I could tell based on the lack of facial expressions and flat tone of voice they were entertaining him long enough to determine whether he was Form 1 eligible' (field notes). That police officers would suspect possible mental health issues when responding to unfounded noise complaints is not surprising given these calls are not entirely uncommon. Encounter 376 is one such example. A male has phoned 9-1-1- reporting 'a male voice cursing and things being smashed. He is not sure where [the noise] is coming from ... It sounds like it is coming from outside, but he can't see anything. He hears a male and female. The female is saying, "Stop! Stop!"' (field notes). Police question neighbours, but no one else has heard anything. They then question the complainant, asking him about his mental health status. He acknowledges having been diagnosed as schizophrenic but denies the possibility that the noises he reported might be auditory hallucinations. Despite the fact none of his neighbours confirm his story, he tells police, '"I'm not crazy ... Other people heard it too this time"' (field notes). In reviewing his record of police interactions, it is clear what he means by 'this time': he has 27 previous 'unfounded' calls, including 6 previous noise complaints.

Potential Victims/Potential Harm

Police also frequently encounter PMI in situations where the individual may be at risk of victimization or of coming to some other form of harm. Encounter 151 illustrates the classic 'social work' response of police officers when dealing with a PMI who is also homeless and has run out of other choices: arresting someone 'for their own good' (Bittner, 1967, 1990). This type of arrest is what researchers have referred to as a 'mercy booking'—a situation in which a vulnerable individual is taken into custody in order to remove them from potential harm and provide basic necessities (Lamb et al., 2002; Wells & Schafer, 2006). Encounter 151 is initiated by a case worker at a local shelter who wants police to remove an intoxicated male. This male has nowhere else to go. He cannot be sent to other facilities because these services lack the staff trained in dealing with someone who is inebriated and has paranoid delusions. Police check, and the local detox centre is also full for the night. Realizing the man will come to some form of harm if they 'make him go on the streets in his current condition' (field notes), they improvise a solution. He is arrested on a charge of public intoxication in order to take him to the lock-up for the night. At the lock-up, the researcher realizes that not only has the arresting officer had many interactions with him, but the 'staff at cell block also appeared to know him well' and he has friendly conversations with several staff members (field notes). Given the state of the man's physical condition, and the potential harm he could have faced being outside in freezing weather in his inebriated state, the researcher notes, the arrest 'is a bit of a blessing for him because the cell is warm, dry and he gets fed' (field notes).

PMI as Suspects or Potential Suspects

Disturbance/Disorderly Conduct

Disturbance calls are typically generated by members of the public and local businesses in response to individuals in obvious distress, acting in ways that provoke suspicion or who are otherwise seen as being disruptive. One such 'suspicious person call' involved a 'regular' who was well known to the attending officer. He is a 32-year-old male sex offender with significant mental health issues. He is presently distraught because he has missed his bus. Police officers locate him walking away from a McDonald's restaurant shouting '"I need help", "I need to go to bed", "I can't keep doing this", "I need to get to work", and "I'm having a panic attack"' (field notes). At first, when the officers arrive, he ignores them. Eventually, they are able to de-escalate the situation by driving him downtown to get a piece of cheesecake.

Disturbance calls initiated by members of the public can also involve vandalism, minor property damage, and/or loud or otherwise obnoxious behaviours that are seen as disruptive to the peace of residents or businesses. Encounter 56 begins with a 9-1-1 call from a local resident who is observing a male overturning recycling bins. She is worried about possible damage to her car, which is parked nearby. As the disturbance is in-progress, the call is dispatched as a Priority 1 call. When police arrive, they discover a 38-year-old Black male, who is upset because he has apparently been trying to get into the building next door. The building is well known to police as a 'drug flop house' (field notes). The man, who is deaf, is asked to produce identification.[1] The officers grow increasingly frustrated officers at the man's inability to produce any identification. Finally, they let him go, despite the fact the upset tenant is adamant that she wants him charged for a criminal offense.

Another call type we have included under the disturbance category is 'unwanted person'—that is, someone whose presence alone is seen as causing a disturbance for a resident or business. In Encounter 171, both the complainant and the 'unwanted person' have mental health issues. According to the complainant, she had befriended a woman she saw as 'lonely', invited her for coffee, and then gave her home address. She then subsequently began experiencing repeated uninvited visits (field notes). The complainant no longer wants this woman visiting and has asked police to make her stop. She also alleges that when she runs into the other woman on the street she is sworn at and called various names. Once the officer ascertains the second woman's identity, he realizes she has a lengthy police history, including *Mental Health Act*-related calls. However, as the threshold for legal charges has not been met, the officer develops a safety plan for the complainant to follow and advises her to call the police when the 'unwanted person' is in her building.

Sometimes mental health issues play a role in neighbourhood disputes. One such dispute involved a woman with mental illness who was engaged in mutually antagonistic clashes with her neighbours. The officer described her as 'doing crazy things' that cause the neighbours to retaliate. However, he was quick to add: 'the neighbours, they're not innocent either. They hate her'. These types of disputes can strain police resources, particularly in smaller communities. In the course of 1 week of conducting fieldwork in the general duty section of a small police station, one of the authors observed multiple calls for service coming in from two sets of neighbours in a local dispute. At one point, the frustrated general duty officer had to yell down the line for the caller to stop screaming and then hung up.

Criminal Suspects

Encounter 104 is a classic example of the type of minor criminal offenses for which PMI are often brought to the attention of police. A homeless shelter calls 9-1-1 to report that one of their clients has been using crystal methamphetamine and has

---

[1] Later another officer, hearing the man's description, supplies his name. He has a lengthy criminal history, and is a suspect for several offenses including, domestic violence, a sexual offense, and gang activity.

been reported to them as having broken into the shed of the mother of another client. Shelter staff advise he cannot return to the shelter because he has been consuming drugs, so they have 'called the cops' (Bittner, 1967). Their expectation is that attending officers will resolve the situation. From the field notes:

> When the staff member came downstairs, she once again told [the] officer that since he is high/tweaking he can't stay. When he told her that was fine because he would be arrested for breach of probation – she wasn't happy about that. [The] officer says, "What does she expect the police are going to do?"

Several decades earlier, Abram and Teplin (1991, p. 1040) observed that in dealing with calls regarding PMI, 'police officers often make the rounds of the various service agencies-receiving rejections from halfway houses, hospitals, and detoxification facilities—before resorting to arrest'. In this instance, the police are starved for choice: the shelter client has told both police and social services he does not want help for his addiction, mental health or other issues, which means most social service agencies will not take him. As a result, the officers use the only option available: as he is in violation of probation conditions, they take him into custody while trying to get him off the streets for a night while they try to come up with a release plan.

Another type of minor offense that results in calls for police service is shoplifting. As we saw in Chap. 1, two calls for service involving PMI in both studies originated from retail stores and involved allegations of 'theft under $5000'. Encounter 340 is one of these cases: it begins with a call from a grocery store involving an allegation of shoplifting. The suspect has purportedly shoplifted dog treats with a dollar value of $2.79. What makes this situation perplexing for the attending officer is the accused has the funds to pay for the item. When police arrive, he has been placed under a citizen's arrest by store security and is agitated and swearing. Despite the fact he has a lengthy criminal history—including as a suspect in 41 domestic violence calls—he is given a warning and released. This response by police is hardly surprising: the potential likelihood of charges being approved by prosecutors is low and, even so, arresting this individual for stolen dog treats will effect zero positive change for the suspect and waste valuable police resources. *Contra* the criminalization hypothesis—the view among some criminologists and members of the public that PMI are disproportionately more likely to be arrested across all offense types (Abramson, 1972; Teplin, 1984; Dempsey et al., 2020)—we see police exercise discretion and make such decisions repeatedly with what they perceive as low-level offenses (see also Engel & Silver, 2001). As Green (1997, p. 483) has observed, 'arrests in nonviolent situations, or issuing citations, are generally considered futile' by most police officers, unless they can be used to achieve some type of objective.

While acts of violence or other forms of major crime by PMI are statistically rare (Watson & Wood, 2017), violence *is* one behaviour that increases the odds someone will initiate a police response. Often such reports are within the context of a domestic dispute, where family members have few other resources available to end the dispute safely or to deal with ongoing issues associated with mental illness (Wood et al., 2021). Encounter 088 was dispatched as a domestic dispute involving a

19-year-old male, who has threatened 'to slit his father's throat if he doesn't give the Internet back to him' (field notes). The young man has no criminal history; however, his mother has previously called the police over 'similar problem behaviour' (field notes). The father describes his son as living with mild Asperger's, Attention Deficit Disorder and depression, but says the son refuses to take his medication, thus leading to family disputes. The father also tells officers he is fearful of his safety and wants the son removed from the house. The officers review the various legal options available and, at the request of the father, he is charged with Uttering Threats and arrested. Aware the real issue is mental health, the officers also consider options for where he can be taken post-release, and the arresting officer includes a recommendation in his charge file that the young man's case be heard in Mental Health court.

Encounter 25 also begins as a domestic dispute. A woman's boyfriend has reported that her 14-year-old daughter has struck her in the back. The woman has fibromyalgia, and the suspect purportedly hit her while she was laying on her bed. From the field notes: 'when the call was dispatched the victim was in hysterics and the daughter had taken her dog for a walk'. The daughter is known to police and has been flagged M for 'mental health'. When she is located and returned, two officers de-escalate the situation before issuing a verbal warning. 'A referral card for Crisis was given to mum and daughter but one is already on the fridge' (field notes).

One aspect of police involvement in responding to PMI calls that has drawn little public attention is the role social service and mental healthcare workers play in initiating police calls regarding acts of violence. Much has been made in media reporting of police-involved shootings and other uses of force involving PMI of the training and skills social workers and psychiatric personnel have in de-escalating violence (Russell, 2020; Donato, 2020). However, what this commentary typically ignores is the research literature (Schwartz & Park, 1999; Allen et al., 2014; Gupta et al., 2018), which has clearly documented the fact that violence by PMI does happen in psychiatric and social work settings, leading to situations in which workers and other clients become the victims of violence. Increasing the odds of police intervention are provincial policies that mandate police involvement in situations where someone's safety is threatened. Encounter 077 begins with an 'assault' call at a provincial group home for youth operated under the authority of Family and Children Services. Following a verbal argument over a TV channel, one youth has 'physically assaulted another youth by punching him in the face' (field notes). Although the alleged suspect is technically 'too old' to be in 'care', he is deemed unable to care for himself as a result of his mental health issues. From the field notes:

> [His] emotional state is very unstable and unpredictable … He is very hard to place because of his maturity level, criminal history, mental instability, and the need to supervise him 24/7. According [to] the group home staff, his mother is an alcoholic and has many other "issues". His most recent statement of intent to commit suicide is by jumping off a bridge. He has also attempted to overdose on his psychotropic medications. [He] reports he experiences auditory and visual hallucinations on a regular basis.

Despite a lengthy history of criminal offenses, previous charges and arrests had clearly made little difference in altering his behaviour or providing him with treatment. Yet, the group home personnel request he be charged and arrested. The rationale for this demand is unclear; however, previous research by Watson and Wood (2017) reveals it is not unusual for complainants to request arrest as a disposition in cases involving PMI. What makes such demands particularly disconcerting is that previous research has demonstrated that the presence or absence of a complainant can influence police decision-making (Patch & Arrigo, 1999), and therefore may contribute significantly to what has been termed the 'criminalization of mental illness' (Abramson, 1972).

Dispatched calls requesting police assistance involving acts of violence at hospitals were also noted during field research. One such call came from the psychiatric ward of a local hospital where a 22-year-old female had assaulted a staff member. As a result of previous encounters with this individual, she had been flagged as both violent and assaultive. Police are advised that 'she wants to be shot by police, so they are to use extra caution' (field notes). The officer with whom the researcher is working alongside explains, 'at a previous call for service she had stated 'Shoot me. Shoot me'. She was walking towards the officers with a knife to her throat while the officers' weapons were drawn' (field notes).

Whereas the majority of police interventions in both studies were the direct result of calls for service, it is the case that some interventions are police-initiated. Another episode of violence involving a PMI was related by a police officer in one of the in-depth interviews conducted for Study 1. This call began as a proactive police-initiated response to observing a crowd of people standing around a fight at a bus shelter. The officer reports seeing 'an old man barely able to walk and he's got a cane and he's beating on a ... 19-year-old kid'. The altercation began when the two men had bumped into each other on the sidewalk. The older man had then retaliated by 'whacking' the younger one (field notes). Bystanders stepped in after the youth responded by punching the older man in the face. While they were holding him, the older man was apparently trying to hit him with his cane. While attempting to resolve the dispute, the officer discovered the young man was dealing with significant mental health issues: 'the kid just happens to be coming out of ... these meetings where these suicidal people get together and they have a counsellor'. A year later, the young man comes to police attention again: 'Unfortunately, that same kid wound up killing a neighbour with a knife about a year later ... Do you remember the one where an old man was giving Christmas cards out and he went over and stabbed him?'

Potential Threats

PMI-related calls also involve situations in which individuals with mental illness are seen as potential threats to others. In some instances, fears might be generated solely from viewing behaviour that is seen as 'odd'; in other instances, police calls are initiated for potentially violent behaviours that generate fears regardless of the actor. In relation to the latter, an incident involving a possible threat of violence begins with a dispatched call from a homeless shelter. A female resident purportedly had a weapon in her backpack—a gun—that she has been waving around. Upon arrival, she is described as 'agitated, arrogant, and belligerent' (field notes). The Emergency Response Unit (ERU) also attends. The weapon turned out to be an imitation firearm. One of the ERU officers tries to de-escalate the situation, so that he can give her a verbal warning. When his attempts fail, she is arrested. While being taken to be processed at the police station, while one of the officers begins making calls to see if an area homeless shelter will accept her upon release—another classic example of proactive problem solving by police officers, who recognize the woman will be a threat to herself or others if she does not have some type of accommodation on release.

Conclusions

In this chapter we examined a diverse array of calls for service related to crime and disorder. *Contra* previous research that has focused near-exclusively on how police-citizen encounters lead to the criminalization of PMI, what we have demonstrated here is that attention also needs to be paid to the ways in which PMI interact with police as victims of crime and as complainants in both crime and disorder-related calls.

As with previous chapters, analysis of calls for service related to crime and disorder are initiated by family, businesses, social service facilities, the general public, and by PMI as both victims and complainants. In relation to the latter, we observed that calls where PMI were complainants were likely to be subsequently cleared as 'unfounded' and/or involved situations where informal warnings were issued. Based on the previous literature, it may be the case—although we have no evidence to support this contention—that PMI who have been victimized are less likely to report crimes to the police for fear of not being believed or due to previous negative interactions (Livingston et al., 2014; Kouyoumdjian et al., 2019).

As with events that we categorized as 'public safety-related', some calls for police service that fall under the umbrella of crime and disorder were initiated in response to 'possible threats'—that is, individuals who were seen to represent potential risks to others. In other words, police are frequently mobilized not because of what someone has done, but because of perceptions of what they might do.

References

Abram, K., & Teplin, L. (1991). Co-occurring disorders among mentally ill jail detainees: Implications for public policy. *American Psychologist, 46*, 1036–1046.

Abramson, M. (1972). The criminalization of mentally disordered behavior: Possible side effect of a new mental health law. *Hospital and Community Psychiatry, 23*, 101–105.

Allen, D., Harris, F., & de Nesnera, A. (2014). Nurse-police coalition: Improves safety in acute psychiatric hospital. *Journal of Psychosocial Nursing and Mental Health Services, 52*(9), 27–31.

References

Bittner, E. (1967). The police on skid-row: A study of peace keeping. *American Sociological Review, 32*(5), 699–715.

Bittner, E. (1990). *Aspects of police work*. Northeastern University Press.

Brink, J., Livingston, J., Desmarais, S., Greaves, C., Maxwell, V., Michalak, E., ... Weaver, C. (2011). *A study of how people with mental illness perceive and interact with the police*. Mental Health Commission of Canada.

Burczyka, M. (2018). *Violent victimization of canadians with mental health-related disabilities, 2014*, Juristat Report: 85-002-x [online]. https://www150.statcan.gc.ca/n1/pub/85-002-x/2018001/article/54977-eng.htm

Charette, Y., Crocker, A. G., & Billette, I. (2014). Police encounters involving citizens with mental illness: Use of resources and outcomes. *Psychiatric Services, 65*(4), 511–516.

Dempsey, C., Quanbeck, C., Bush, C., & Kruger, K. (2020). Decriminalizing mental illness: Specialized policing responses. *CNS Spectrums, 25*(2), 181–195.

Donato, A. (2020). How to de-escalate a mental health emergency without calling the police. *The Huffington Post*. https://www.huffingtonpost.ca/entry/deescalate-mental-health-crisis-tips_ca_5ef67d60c5b6ca97090fa2b1

Engel, R., & Silver, E. (2001). Policing mentally disordered subjects: A re-examination of the criminalization hypothesis. *Criminology, 39*, 225–252.

Frederick, T., O'Connor, C., & Koziarski, J. (2018). Police interactions with people perceived to have a mental health problem: A critical review of frames, terminology, and definitions. *Victims & Offenders, 13*(8), 1037–1054.

Green, T. (1997). Police as frontline mental health workers. The decision to arrest or refer to mental health agencies. *International Journal of Law & Psychiatry, 20*(4), 469–486.

Gupta, S., Akyuz, E., Flint, J., & Baldwin, T. (2018). Violence and aggression in psychiatric settings: Reporting to the police. *British Journal Psychiatry Advances, 24*(3), 146–151.

Huey, L. (2007). *Negotiating demands: The politics of skid row policing in Edinburgh, San Francisco, and Vancouver*. University of Toronto Press.

Huey, L., & Broll, R. (2018). *Becoming strong: Impoverished women and the struggle to overcome violence*. University of Toronto Press.

Kouyoumdjian, F., Wang, R., Mejia-Lancheros, C., Owusu-Bempah, A., Nisenbaum, R., et al. (2019). Interactions between police and persons who experience homelessness and mental illness in Toronto, Canada: Findings from a prospective study. *Canadian Journal of Psychiatry, 64*(10), 718–725.

Lamb, H., Weinberger, L., & DeCuir, W. (2002). The police and mental health. *Psychiatric Services, 53*(10), 1266–1271.

Livingston, J., Desmarais, S., Greaves, C., Parent, R., Verdun-Jones, S., & Brink, J. (2014). What influences perceptions of procedural justice among people with mental illness regarding their interactions with the police? *Community Mental Health Journal, 50*(3), 281–287.

Patch, P., & Arrigo, B. (1999). Police officer attitudes and use of discretion in situations involving the mentally ill: The need to narrow the focus. *International Journal of Law and Psychiatry, 22*(1), 23–35.

Russell, T. (2020). Social workers are masters at de-escalation. Here's what the police can learn from them. *The Week*. https://theweek.com/articles/926513/social-workers-are-masters-deescalation-heres-what-police-learn-from

Schulenberg, J. (2016). Police decision-making in the gray zone: The dynamics of police–citizen encounters with mentally ill persons. *Criminal Justice and Behavior, 43*(4), 459–482.

Schwartz, T., & Park, T. (1999). Assaults by patients on psychiatric residents: A survey and training recommendations. *Psychiatric Services, 50*(3), 381–383.

Shore, K., & Lavoie, J. (2019). Exploring mental health-related calls for police service: A Canadian study of police officers as 'frontline mental health workers'. *Policing: A Journal of Policy and Practice, 13*(2), 157–171.

Teplin, L. (1984). Criminalizing mental disorder: The comparative arrest rate of the mentally ill. *American Psychologist, 39*(7), 794–803.

Teplin, L., McClelland, G., Abram, K., & Weiner, D. (2005). Crime victimization in adults with severe mental illness: Comparison with the National Crime Victimization Survey. *Archives of General Psychiatry, 62*(8), 911–921.

Watson, A., & Wood, J. D. (2017). Everyday police work during mental health encounters: A study of call resolutions in Chicago and their implications for diversion. *Behavioral Sciences & the Law, 35*(5–6), 442–455.

Wells, W., & Schafer, J. (2006). Officer perceptions of police responses to persons with a mental illness. *Policing: An International Journal of Police Strategies & Management, 29*(4), 578–601.

Wood, J., Watson, A., & Barber, C. (2021). What can we expect of police in the face of deficient mental health systems? Qualitative insights from Chicago police officers. *Journal of Psychiatric and Mental Health Nursing, 28*(1), 28–42.

Chapter 4
Police Attitudes Towards Their Roles in Dealing with Mental Health Issues

In this chapter, we draw extensively on both interview data and research field notes to explore how officers see police work in relation to mental health calls. What our analysis reveals is that some 50 plus years after Bittner's (1967, 1974) groundbreaking work on the intersection of frontline policing and mental health, police work continues to be significantly impacted by mental health-related calls, with officers continuing to serve as informal gatekeepers to the mental health system. For the officers Bittner observed, serving in this capacity was seen as a source of social work that frustrates their ability to engage in law enforcement, famously captured in his conceptualization of policing as 'Florence Nightingale in Pursuit of Willie Sutton' (Bittner, 1974). The officers observed in our studies were also frequently frustrated; however, as we document in the pages below, the source of their frustration is with a worsening mental health system and their frequent inability to paper over its cracks.

Is Mental Health a Significant Policing Issue?

> Researcher: So mental health, is that a problem?
> Police Officer: Absolutely!

Over 60 years of research has consistently documented several facts about policing and PMI. The first we address is the police view that mental health issues are a significant driver of calls for service (Bittner, 1967; Teplin, 1984; Patch & Arrigo, 1999; Wells & Schafer, 2006; Coleman & Cotton, 2014; Gatens, 2018; see also de-Tribolet Hardy et al., 2015). The second is the perception that these calls consume significant police resources relative to many other call types (Short et al., 2014; Griffiths et al., 2015; Rhodes, 2018). The findings from our research are no different. With only one exception, which we discuss shortly, police officers across both studies expressed the belief that, as one officer said, 'mental health is a huge, huge issue [in police work]'.

Officers interviewed for Study 1 saw mental health as not only a major factor in calls involving adults, but also among youth. One officer who works with young people in the local school system stated, 'I'm finding a nexus between mental health and drug use, mental health and depression, and the cutting themselves and that sort of thing'. Another stated, 'I did a lot of arrests on the road, all mental health'. His view on the prevalence of mental health issues among detained youth was shaped, he said, by asking young people about the type of medications they were on while filling out 'detain sheets'. '"Yes, I'm on medication" Anxiety disorders, ADHD, ADD, um what's the one? Oppositional defiance disorder, that's the big one that they all have. They all have something'. A frontline officer in another area of the service said of dealing with youth, 'a good chunk of my time is spent with mental health', young people who are often reported missing because 'they don't go home'. During ride-alongs, officers expressed similar views. Frontline patrol is seen as comprising a lot of well-being checks, suicide, and other mental health-related calls. With each of these, comes the possibility that officers will spend their entire shift 'babysitting' (Bittner, 1990).

Over the course of interviews, and in comments made during field observations, officers offered a number of explanations for what they see as the prevalence of mental health issues both generally, and in relation to their work. One explained it as a result of poor diets, particularly for young people: 'I believe that a lot of ... children are growing up lacking nutrients in their development and it's affecting their brain'. Others questioned whether changes in diagnostic practices were playing a role: 'I would like someone to find for me what are the reasons behind the rise in mental illness and anxiety issues and disorders in children and young adults? That wasn't there 30 years ago or was there and it just wasn't diagnosed?' Family dysfunction is another cited cause, along with drug abuse. 'I think obviously the drugs would lead to mental health issues ... or at least like a psychosis type situation when it comes to that,' one explained. Similarly, an officer from another area of the same city offered the following opinion: 'I think that we're very fragile and when we're putting drugs into our system, you know, just for the highs and stuff like that, we often [wind] up with imbalances'. Only one officer felt differently, in that he attributed the bulk of crime and disorder-related calls solely to addiction. From the fieldnotes:

> Contrary to other officers that I have spoken to, this officer does not believe that the majority of the calls that he attends are mental health related. He stated that the biggest issue that he has come across are drugs.

Should Mental Health Be 'Police Property'?

In analysing both the observational notes and interview data, one of the questions we sought to answer was whether, or to what extent, police officers felt that mental health *should* be 'police property'. In our work with police agencies across Canada, we have certainly heard differences in opinion among officers on this same question. For instance, one senior police leader in major metropolitan police service privately expressed to one of us that the possibility of violence at many mental health calls makes him a believer in the need for a police response. Other officers, and perhaps not surprisingly many of them in frontline patrol work, have publicly or otherwise expressed the view that many of the mental health-related calls they attend should be diverted to crisis units or other agencies, or better still proactively prevented through community initiatives. Perhaps not surprisingly then, we found similar mixed views within our own data.

While none of the officers in either study felt that mental health should never be a police concern, they did differ in their views as to the extent to which different types of calls and related procedures should be undertaken by police. Before examining the majority opinion, it is worth considering one outlier: an officer who felt that 'too much time is spent on responding to 903 [suicide] calls for service'. Clearly frustrated, and possibly burnt out, this officer expressed the view that some people 'are worthwhile to save and others are not' (field notes). He then provided several examples of people he had reached out to help. These examples included the story of a young woman who had had significant issues with drugs and self-harming. With some help, she had gone on to become a university student who was 'doing very well'. But others were seen as having no desire to help themselves, so 'why should we continue to expend resources on them?' As will be seen in the further detail in the next section, frustration was a recurring theme. Whereas the previous officer was frustrated by people's behaviours, in some instances, an individual's views were clearly tied to frustrations with the healthcare system. Another officer among many was 'frustrated' with the lack of accountability among mental health service providers for those clients who abscond or, in the case of voluntary admissions, grow tired of waiting at the hospital and leave. In both such cases, the response is simply to call police to locate and return them—the 'free taxi service' previously mentioned. For these officers, their opinion was their role in dealing with PMI would be greatly reduced if other actors in the system were not so quick to absolve themselves of responsibility for their clients.

Another recurring theme in relation to this question was evidenced by the perspective we have termed, 'if police don't do it, nobody will'. For some officers this perspective entails seeing themselves as frontline 'gatekeepers' to resources that individuals and families in crisis need, but have difficulties accessing or navigating. Encounter 275 illustrates the role that some officers have come to play in this regard. A police officer was notified by dispatch that an individual he had previously arrested was being released from the psychiatric ward at the hospital. Before the man left, the officer had to drive to the hospital to serve him with papers to appear in court. From the field notes:

> The officer explained to the individual the nature of his charges and that he was giving him a promise to appear. He then began to ask the individual if he was getting in touch with any community support groups. #275 stated that he has made contact with various groups and has spoken to his Dad about going to a rehabilitation facility. He said that he wanted to take control of his life and wanted kick his addiction once and for all.

The officer explained to him that he did not want to see him behind bars in jail and wanted him to explain to the crown attorney the steps that he was taking to better himself. The officer seemed genuinely concerned with #275's health and safety. He suggested that he move out of his house – a previously known area for drug abusers and try to spend time with people who can have a positive impact on his life. We then left the room and made our way back to the car.

The officer noted that individuals with MH issues oftentimes 'fall through the cracks' when they are not set up with support services in the community. He said that the individual that we dealt with is in fact one of those people who fell through the cracks. However, he has high hopes for this individual if he takes advantage of community resources.

This police gatekeeping function has more recently been formally institutionalized across several Canadian cities in the form of a programme aimed at developing collaborative risk assessment and resource sharing between police, social service, healthcare, and educational groups of individuals deemed as 'high risk'. Variously known as Situation Tables or Community Hubs, the goal is to identify 'frequent fliers'—that is individuals frequently cycling in and out of the criminal justice system—and to divert them to necessary resources to reduce or remove those risk factors associated with their criminal offending. That said, it is also worth noting that, here too, police express frustration with the decision-making of other institutions and actors. In one of the studies, several officers referred to the case of a mentally ill, homeless male with 112 prior contacts with police, including contacts with at least three different police agencies. In other words, the exact type of individual this collaborative system was designed to assist. When his file was brought forward to the 'Table', other services did not deem the case as sufficiently worthy of action, and so no further action was taken.

A recurring issue raised not only in private conversation with police officers, but also in some media reporting and public responses to high profile cases in the news, is the notion that police need to be involved in mental health-related calls out of safety concerns for PMI and/or members of the public. In both studies, this was not a commonly cited view; however, one officer did raise the issue. This was framed by the officer not as a matter of some interactions with PMI possibly involving violence, but as a concern arising out of real and perceived failures of the mental health system. We see this concern below in an excerpt from an interview:

Officer: Schizophrenia and stuff like that. And now the question is how to deal with them. So we got somebody that's behaving in a way where they … might hurt themselves or others, setting fires at their home or something like that. We'll arrest them under the *Mental Health Act* and take them.

Researcher: But will you also lay the criminal charge as well?

Officer: Well, it depends. The first instance I gave you if there's a criminal charge we'll lay that and let the courts send them to the [mental health court or facility].

Researcher: Ok, but if an act is occurring that is not in contravention of the *Criminal Code* … you'll use the *Mental Health Act*?

Officer: That's right, yeah. And sometimes those acts are criminal. We get people that are waiving knives around, they're cutting themselves. But it's clearly a mental issue, but if they've hurt somebody? Here's the problem … and this happens fairly often, a psychiatrist says, "nope he's not crazy he's just…" and they let him out. But he's been waiving at, you know, he's running after people with a knife.

In other words, the police role in dealing with threats or actual violence was attributed to the inability or unwillingness of mental health providers to perform their ascribed role. In these instances, not only is there an immediate safety concern for police to address, but also the question of how to prevent future harm from someone who might be returned to the public only hours after having been in a potentially dangerous state.

The Impact of These Calls on Officers

In previous sections, we examined what police officers *believe* about their role vis-à-vis mental health. In this section, we explore how they *feel* about these calls—an equally important aspect to understanding how best to move forward in terms of public policy. One of the recurring themes in some public dialogue on policing and mental health has been the notion that police have commandeered the field of public responses to mental health crises—thus diverting money from the public health sector—in order to increase police budgets and justify additional members. Our research among frontline officers documents a very different set of perspectives, from empathy to a frustration that sometimes seemed to border on helplessness.

While some officers were clearly frustrated by mental health calls and, in some instances obviously burnt out, most tended to be empathetic, even, as we have seen in previous chapters, in situations in which their patience was being tested. One of the individuals with whom police in Site 2 routinely interact was described as someone who 'doesn't always understand what is going on around him and the public has little tolerance for him because his constant chatter and lack of volume control scares them' (field notes). One of the officers states he 'feels so bad for this male' and he and his partner worry about 'whether he has any food or if he has access to any services at all' (field notes). Because he is not engaged in any criminal or other activity, and his behaviour likely would not meet the threshold for psychiatric admission, there's little they feel they can do to help him.

A recurring theme in both our data and in the research literature is officer frustration (Godfredson et al., 2011; Simpson, 2015; Wood et al., 2017). For some, it is frustration with what are perceived to be impractical policies that waste their time and police resources. The practice of psychiatric facilities calling police to report 'missing patients' is one such example. When one such call came in, an officer observed, that the hospitals reports the person as missing long after they had already absconded. Hearing similar complaints from others, the researcher notes, 'he isn't the only officer frustrated by this trend'. Among sources of frustration, officers in both studies also cited hours waiting in admissions with PMI and the feeling that such cases were not a priority. Some complained about 'having their entire shift [being] taken up 'babysitting' until [the PMI can be] seen by medical staff, to the point where a relief officer is needed at the end of their shift' (field notes). Similarly, another officer stated, 'we have a lot of problems with working it out with the hospitals where they keep an officer. When we arrest somebody under the *Mental*

Health Act, we tend to sit with them 5–6 h before they'll form them, and we lose an officer for that long'. As a consequence of such long wait times, police services across Canada are increasingly developing protocols with local hospitals to expedite such cases with varied results. Through our other research, we have heard from several different services that such protocols have been highly effective when followed, but are not always followed, causing increasing wait times.

Another source of frustration identified through observation and interview data are repeat 'unfounded' calls made by PMI. As we saw in the previous chapter, individuals experiencing visual or auditory hallucinations may contact police to report noises, fighting or other safety issues necessitating a police response, only to have police investigate and clear the call as 'unfounded'. One woman was repeatedly advised by officers to stop calling the police to remove her son from her home, as he was not engaged in any criminal conduct. The Patrol Sergeant for the area even admonished his officers at parade on the necessity of impressing this information upon her the next time she called. Another PMI had conditions placed upon her to not call emergency services unless the situation was a bona fide emergency. Of this individual, an officer stated in frustration, "She was a nightmare."

Sometimes it is difficult to delineate one theme from another, because they can often be intertwined. This issue was found to be particularly the case in relation to frustration and empathy—sometimes officers were frustrated because of the detrimental impacts to PMI of systemic failures, failures in programmes, and systems designed to help them. Such was the case with programmes such as Situation Tables or Hub models that are ostensibly aimed at improving access to resources for those PMI who are chronically cycling through the criminal justice system, but that frequently deny those resources to individuals who through the criminal justice system but can also fail those individuals. We referenced such a situation earlier in this chapter, with the example of the individual who was deemed by other agencies as not sufficiently 'at risk'. Another source of frustration was with the ability to get cases before the Table in a timely manner. One woman, who was seen as an 'ideal candidate' for the Situation Table by one of the officers in Study 1, died from suicide not long after she was last seen by that officer, walking at night near a cemetery, talking to herself.

More often, though, failures were attributed to the mental health system, which police variously saw as under-resourced and/or dysfunctional. For example, an Officer in Study 2 observed that the local 'psych ward is … not big enough. They can bring someone in on a Form 1 apprehension, but if the ward is full, that's it, regardless of the state of affairs' (field notes). Another officer from this service, complained that PMI would leave one city—with greater resources for individuals with complex needs—and migrate to smaller towns, like his, that had far fewer resources. These migrations were putting strains on not only local police, but also on the mental health resources available. One consistent theme across data from both sites was the view that hospitals maintain too high a threshold for admitting psychiatric cases, with the result that PMI in crisis were being left with too few, if any, resources. One officer complained that he had brought in several individuals who had attempted suicide, only to discover they were subsequently released. From the field notes:

> Within 2-3 days after release, they successfully committed suicide. This is not the first officer I have heard this from. All of the officers understandably have strong emotions about this, whether they are overt about it or not. I always get detailed examples that I am consciously not including in the field notes out of respect for the deceased.

A final frustration documented had to do with police protocols surrounding dropped 9-1-1 calls. An officer complained that, despite the fact these are Priority 1 calls in his service, service protocol does not allow officers to breach the premises to check well-being if no one answers. This officer raised an interesting point: 'what if the person is unconscious?' (field notes).

Compassion fatigue is a common response among individuals who are constantly exposed to conditions that might normally generate an empathetic response. We are not alone in making this observation: numerous studies have documented the prevalence of this form of secondary trauma among police officers (Papazoglou et al., 2019; Burnett et al., 2020). We have already cited one example in this chapter of someone possibly experiencing burnout and, as a result shifting his views of who is and is not worthy of his compassion. Another such example was an officer in Study 2 who told the researcher, he was 'starting to hate 937 [mental health] calls'. That some officers would become irritated, frustrated, and/or burnt out over time in dealing with often complex and potentially volatile situations is not unique to officers in our sample. Research in Germany has documented similar results, showing that police interactions with PMI are often fraught with anxiety for the individual police officer (Wittmann et al., 2020). Other factors that contribute additional challenge and complexity for officers is the level of verbal and physical abuse to which they may be subjected (ibid.). The bulk of encounters reported on here did not involve physical force, with the exception of the one documented case in which an individual bit and hit officers. That said, we did document many situations in which officers were variously screamed at, cursed, lied to, and/or spoken to in an aggressive manner.

Conclusions

For police officers, mental health-related issues remain a significant driver of police calls for service, a factor that many see as increasing in volume. Such a finding is hardly surprising; previous other studies have identified similar results (Coleman & Cotton, 2014). Where this chapter departs from earlier work is in relation to the question of whether officers feel that mental health calls *should* be a police concern. Analysis of both interview and observational data suggests that while none of the frontline officers in either study felt that mental health should never be a police concern, most felt that their involvement should be more focused on cases involving real or potential violence. Interestingly, in some key aspects, their views mirror those of police reformers: both groups feel that a critical examination of what police do and why in this area is necessary.

Although there are some areas of congruence between police and reformer perspectives on the issue of police involvement in mental health calls, there is also a key difference: police officers are the ones being mobilized to prop up what is seen as a failing mental health care system. The awareness of this use, coupled with the inability to effect meaningful change, creates frustration for many. Whereas some are able to hang onto their empathy and compassion, for others, frustration can lead to burnout and/or compassion fatigue. This fact, we argue, remains under-recognized in both the academic literature and in police policy and practice.

References

Bittner, E. (1967). The police on skid-row: A study of peace keeping. *American Sociological Review, 32*(5), 699–715.
Bittner, E. (1974). Florence nightingale in pursuit of willie Sutton: A theory of the police. In H. Jacob (Ed.), *The potential for reform of criminal justice*. Sage.
Bittner, E. (1990). *Aspects of police work*. Northeastern University Press.
Burnett, M., Sheard, I., & St. Clair-Thompson, H. (2020). The prevalence of compassion fatigue, compassion satisfaction and perceived stress, and their relationships with mental toughness, individual differences and number of self-care actions in a UK police force. *Police Practice and Research, 21*(4), 383–400.
Coleman, T., & Cotton, F. (2014). *TEMPO: Police interactions a report towards improving interactions between police and people living with mental health problems*. Report of the Mental Health Commission of Canada. www.mentalhealthcommission.ca
de-Tribolet Hardy, F., Kesic, D., & Thomas, S. (2015). Police management of mental health crisis situations in the community: Status quo, current gaps and future directions. *Policing and Society, 25*(3), 294–307.
Gatens, A. (2018). *Law enforcement response to mental health crisis incidents: A survey of Illinois Police and Sheriff's Departments*. https://icjia.illinois.gov/researchhub/files/MHCR_Article_121318-191011T20093000.pdf
Godfredson, J., Thomas, S., Ogloff, J., & Luebbers, S. (2011). Police perceptions of their encounters with individuals experiencing mental illness: A Victorian survey. *Australian & New Zealand Journal of Criminology, 44*(2), 180–195.
Griffiths, C., Murphy, J., & Tatz, M. (2015). *Improving police efficiency - Challenges and opportunities*. Public Safety Canada Research Report: 2015–R021. https://www.publicsafety.gc.ca/cnt/rsrcs/pblctns/2015-r021/2015-r021-en.pdf
Papazoglou, K., Koskelainen, M., & Stuewe, N. (2019). Examining the relationship between personality traits, compassion satisfaction, and compassion fatigue among police officers. *SAGE Open*. https://doi.org/10.1177/2158244018825190
Patch, P., & Arrigo, B. (1999). Police officer attitudes and use of discretion in situations involving the mentally ill: The need to narrow the focus. *International Journal of Law and Psychiatry, 22*(1), 23–35.
Rhodes, B. (2018). '*Multiagency review of mental health crisis services' in Lincolnshire*. https://www.lincolnshire.gov.uk/downloads/file/2614/lincs-review-of-mental-health-crisis-services-pdfa
Short, T., Macdonald, C., Luebbers, S., Ogloff, J., & Thomas, S. (2014). The nature of police involvement in mental health transfers. *Police Practice and Research, 5*(4), 336–348.
Simpson, J. (2015). Police and homeless outreach worker partnerships: Policing of homeless individuals with mental illness in Washington, D.C. *Human Organization, 74*(2), 125–134.

References

Teplin, L. (1984). Criminalizing mental disorder: The comparative arrest rate of the mentally ill. *American Psychologist, 39*(7), 794–803.

Wells, W., & Schafer, J. (2006). Officer perceptions of police responses to persons with a mental illness. *Policing: An International Journal of Police Strategies & Management, 29*(4), 578–601.

Wittmann, L., Jörns-Presentati, A., & Groen, G. (2020). How do police officers experience interactions with people with mental illness? *Journal of Police and Criminal Psychology, 36*, 220–226.

Wood, J., Watson, A., & Fulambarker, A. (2017). The "gray zone" of police work during mental health encounters: Findings from an observational study in Chicago. *Police Quarterly, 20*(1), 81–105.

Chapter 5
At the Crossroads

Following the death of Mr. George Floyd in Minneapolis on May 25, 2020, citizens across various countries began to demand changes in public policing. Many of these demands coalesced under the slogan, 'defund the police'. In some instances, as we have noted in relation to the death of Ms. Korchinski-Paquet, 'defund the police' became synonymous for many with the idea of diverting portions of police funding to mental health and social work responses for responding to individuals in crisis and/or with mental illnesses. Throughout this book, however, we have attempted to show the myriad of ways in which public policing has become entangled in mental health issues and some of the complexities surrounding the roles they are called upon to play. More specifically, across public safety and crime/disorder domains, we show that PMI can become 'police property' in a variety of roles—as a victim, complainant, or the subject of a complaint—and that the police are be mobilized to PMI in the community by a multitude of different actors, such as family, friends, or even the PMI themselves. In some cases, we even observe the police being mobilized to situations involving PMI by social service and hospital staff—the very group of people that some reformers would like to see take the place of the police in responding to mental health issues in the community. This particular finding highlights the complexities around disentangling mental health from the police mandate if the police are being mobilized, in some circumstances, by the very people reformer have slated to replace them.

A further complexity that we identify is that while some of the ways in which PMI become 'police property' are very evident in that they can or may involve a mental health component, such a mental health calls, attempted suicide calls, or wellness checks, other reasons for police mobilization may not reveal that PMI are involved until after the police are on scene. Recall, for example, the traffic-related incident that we discussed in Chap. 2. In these circumstances it would be impossible to know from the onset as to whether a non-police mental health response would be needed as the call came in for something that is very clearly part of the police mandate. Furthermore, we also observe that, in some circumstances, the nature of the police mobilization can dynamically change. For instance, we provide examples where calls initially dispatched for returning PMI to hospital or suicide threats are subsequently changed to high-priority missing persons investigations—a role of the police mandate that also has not been up for debate as part of the 'defund the police' movement.

In sum, our findings point to not only the myriad of ways that mental health has become 'police property', but the immense complexity around disentangling mental health from the police mandate. Indeed, as some of our interview participants alluded to in the previous chapter, there is a need to fix existing upstream solutions that have, for a variety of reasons, been failing thus forcing the police to step into fill-in the cracks. However, given the myriad of ways that PMI become police property, along with the fact that no upstream solution will be 100% effective, it is pertinent that the police continue to be prepared for encountering PMI in their daily activities. In light of this, we discuss some possible upstream and downstream policy and practice solutions which may not only serve to reduce the footprint of the police in the lives of PMI more generally but can help narrow the role of the police in circumstances where they may be needed.

Upstream Solutions

The first, but perhaps most requested and discussed solution to reduce the footprint of the police in the lives of PMI is to adequately fund hospital- and community-based mental health care. As has been well documented elsewhere, the deinstitutionalization of PMI in the 1970s was intended to occur in tandem with the establishing of mental health supports for PMI in the community (Lamb & Bachrach, 2001; Lamb et al., 2002). While *some* supports were indeed established post-deinstitutionalization, the breadth of mental health care—as well as the funding directed towards mental health care—has always been perceived as a policy failure on the part of governments. Even now, approximately five decades post-deinstitutionalization, we continue to witness how low of a priority mental health care is to many governments. Our home province of Ontario, Canada for example—the most populace province in the country—only spends approximately 7% of healthcare funding toward mental health (Lurie, 2014). This lack of mental health care, as well as funding toward expanding care, has inevitably generated numerous consequences for PMI which in turn push some toward coming into contact with the police. Perhaps most evidently, a lack of accessible mental health care means that there are likely many living in the community with undiagnosed or untreated mental illness because they simply cannot get the care that they require. When or if these individuals reach crisis, the police may be put in a position to respond. Indeed, as many of our interview participants identified within the previous chapter, they perceive the police as propping up an under-resourced and dysfunctional mental health system. On the other hand, those who *do* opt to navigate the underfunded mental health system can face wait times for care that can stretch months, if not years

(Children's Mental Health Ontario, 2020; Goldner et al., 2011). These long wait times can leave unaddressed problems to escalate, and in some instances, to the point of a mental health crises thus, again, instigating a police response.

When police do respond, as we have seen in previous chapters, the lack of mental health care can also have implications for them and their interactions with PMI. For example, a lack of hospital beds for psychiatric patients can mean that, in some instances, when a PMI is transported to hospital by police, the individual in question may not be admitted simply because the hospital may not have the room to take the individual in and/or room is reserved only for the most serious of cases (Koziarski et al., 2020). Such situations—as alluded to by our study participants—sustain what has come to be known as the 'revolving door' of the mental health system, whereby individuals are taken to hospital with the hope that they will be assessed and admitted into treatment. Instead, they are released, only to come into contact with the police once again a short time later (Canada et al., 2010; Iacobucci, 2014; Markowitz, 2011). Unfortunately, some situations involving a released individual, as we described in the previous chapter, can lead to a tragic end.

Undoubtedly, having an adequately funded and fully accessible mental health system can not only lead to PMI securing the care that they require, but by doing so, can also reduce the footprint of the police in the lives of PMI across many of the ways in which PMI become police property. That said, however, we do also believe that an accessible mental health system is not a panacea as there are other pertinent steps that can be taken, in tandem with enhancing mental health care accessibility, that can ensure an even further reduced police footprint. Other avenues, for instance, include addressing issues around homelessness and substance use. It is believed that providing PMI experiencing homelessness with sustainable and/or supportive housing can reduce the psychological and physical stresses of homelessness, while creating opportunities to adequately address issues around their mental health (Koziarski et al., 2020; Huey & Broll, 2018; Padgett et al., 2011). This is also the case for PMI with substance use issues. Studies have previously found that the co-occurrence of mental illness and substance use is not uncommon for interactions between PMI and police (Charette et al., 2011; Shore & Lavoie, 2019), and thus by addressing any possible issues around substance use, it is believed that it can provide an opportunity for the individual to address their mental illness while not simultaneously navigating substance use (Harris & Edlund, 2005). Indeed, some PMI may also be experiencing homelessness and substance use disorder simultaneously, which only exacerbates barriers toward successful mental health treatment (Kirst et al., 2015; Padgett et al., 2011). Although, as we elaborate upon shortly, should these (and other) solutions be enacted as a means to reduce the footprint of the police in the lives of PMI, it is crucial that such efforts are continuously evaluated to ensure that they are successfully achieving this outcome.

Beyond system-level changes, we also believe that it is fruitful to explore individual- or family-level approaches, as well. Work by Watson and Wood (2017) and others (e.g., Charette et al., 2011; Teplin & Pruett, 1992) have found that most interactions between police and PMI conclude with no action on the part of officers because there are no legal grounds to arrest the individual or apprehend them under mental health legislation—otherwise referred to as the 'grey zone' of police-PMI interactions. This, Watson and Wood (2017) argue, points toward the possibility of broadening existing pre-arrest diversion efforts—some of which we will discuss in the subsequent section—so that the police are not the sole stakeholders attempting to divert PMI away from the criminal justice system (see also Schulenberg, 2016). For instance, many of the examples of police-PMI interactions that we provided within the previous chapters were—at least in-part—preceded by a lack of medication adherence. As such, Watson and Wood (2017) suggest that options such as post-emergency room follow-up and family engagement could ensure the individual's continued engagement in mental health care and adherence to prescribed medications, which could lessen the chance of a mental health crisis and thus police involvement.

Moreover, the fact that most interactions between police and PMI occur in this 'grey zone', points toward an opportunity to possibly remove the police as responders to *some* PMI calls altogether. In other words, calls which are explicitly reported as being primarily mental health-related in nature could receive a civilian-based response that is comprised of crisis workers or other mental health professionals. Such efforts are already underway in jurisdictions such as Eugene, Oregon where Crisis Assistance Helping Out on the Streets (CAHOOTS)—a civilian team comprised of a crisis worker and a medic—has been the primary response to mental health calls since 1989 (White Bird Clinic, 2020). Of the approximately 24,000 calls that CAHOOTS responded to in 2019, police assistance was requested at 150 of those calls (White Bird Clinic, 2020).

Further potential opportunities to reduce the footprint of the police in the lives of PMI are being offered through emerging work that focuses on the spatial patterns of interactions with PMI. More specifically, a growing body of research has shown that mental health calls to the police cluster spatially (Vaughan et al., 2016, 2018; White & Goldberg, 2018; Hodgkinson & Andresen, 2019; Koziarski, 2020). In light of this, some scholars have made the case for reorienting police-led, pre-arrest diversion efforts to proactively focus on hot spots of where interactions between the police and PMI occur most frequently as doing so may mitigate the need for future police involvement in crisis scenarios (Koziarski, 2020; White & Weisburd, 2017). Another strategy, further upstream than the police, would be for cities to use this and other forms of data analysis to improve identification of individuals in crisis and provide appropriate street outreach and support from social workers and healthcare professionals, as is already occurring in some major cities.

While each of the ideas above represent promising upstream methods of reducing the footprint of the police in the lives of PMI, the complexity around the myriad of ways that PMI become police property—that is, police mobilizations which may not be immediately evident that they involve PMI or mobilizations that can dynamically change—points to the fact that we can only *reduce* the footprint of the police in the lives of PMI, not completely *eliminate* it (see also Ratcliffe, 2021). As such, it is paramount that the police not only continue to be prepared for responding to PMI in the community, but are also aware of steps that they can possibly take to reduce their footprint in the lives of PMI.

Downstream Solutions

Once again, because police-PMI interactions often occur in a grey zone where officers do not have the legal authority to arrest nor apprehend an individual under mental health legislation, officers should be informed on potential steps that they can take at the culmination of these encounters that could serve toward reducing their footprint in the lives of PMI. Admittedly, options are relatively limited in these particular instances. However, one potentially helpful approach would be for officers to have a thorough understanding of local, community-based mental health resources (Watson & Wood, 2017). This would include not only knowing where such resources are located or their hours of operation, but also potentially having hard-copy materials on hand from the nearest resource that can be given to the individual or their families so that they can be informed on the services that they have close by. Officers could also potentially offer to transport the individual in question to the location should they be willing while in the presence of responding officers. Indeed, while offering to transport PMI to resources at the culmination of an interaction may appear as though the police are *increasing* their footprint, the potential long-term outcome is that engagement with mental health resources—particularly sustained engagement—could prevent said individual from coming into contact with police in the future.

Another potential avenue through which the police could reduce their footprint in the lives of PMI is to increase their competency around whether or not to apprehend someone under the *Mental Health Act*. Research comparing outcomes of interactions with PMI between frontline officers and co-response teams—that is, specialized responses to mental health calls which are comprised of a specially trained officer and a mental health practitioner—show that co-response teams reduce unnecessary hospital transfers relative to frontline-only responses (Fahim et al., 2016; Semple et al., 2020). Indeed, having a mental health practitioner at the scene of co-response interactions improves the decision-making as to whether or not to take someone to hospital for an assessment, but having frontline officers improve their skills on this front can not only prevent unnecessary transfers but it can also save officers needlessly waiting in an emergency room for the hospital to take custody of—and subsequently release—someone who may have not needed to come to the hospital in the first place. As alluded to in Chap. 1, one possible avenue through which officer decision-making could be assisted on this front is the adoption of frontline mental health screeners (Hirdes et al., 2019; Hoffman et al., 2016). HealthIM (n.d.), for example, is a digitized version of the interRAI Brief Mental Health Screener which is constructed of a 14-variable algorithm that, according to Hoffman et al. (2016), has been tested to accurately determine who was most likely to be transported to hospital by officers, and who was most likely to be admitted into the hospital. Officers spend approximately 4–5 min answering questions on the screener based on what the officer is observing from the individual (e.g., actions, symptoms, etc.), as well as what is said from bystanders and caretakers. Once the screener is completed, HealthIM (n.d.) runs a risk analysis and provides the officer(s) with scores out of ten related risk of harm to self, risk of harm to others, and self-care in order to allow officers to make a more informed decision as to whether or not to take the individual to hospital for assessment.

For situations where taking individuals to hospital *is* appropriate, the police should strive to establish transfer agreements between themselves and the facility so that PMI are transferred into the care of the hospital in a timelier manner. As we have described earlier, and as other studies have similarly found, a considerable portion of an officer's shift can be consumed with waiting for a PMI to be transferred into the custody of the hospital (Iacobucci, 2014; Wells & Schafer, 2006). Agreements that are put in place and adhered to could minimize the footprint of the police in the lives of PMI by reducing the amount of time that police spend with PMI to begin with, which could also free up costly police resources. Some co-response teams and other pre-arrest diversion efforts—such as Crisis Intervention Teams (CIT) which are comprised of officers who received extensive training on mental health—already have such agreements in place (Iacobucci, 2014; Steadman et al., 2001), but it would be worthwhile exploring the extension of such agreements to *all* police transfers to the hospital since frontline officers do attend more mental health calls than co-response efforts (Iacobucci, 2014).

Another potential avenue through which the footprint of the police in the lives of PMI could be reduced is through the expansion of efforts such as CIT and co-response. Not only can such efforts lead to additional benefits when it comes to police-PMI interactions more generally, such as reduced arrest or use of force (Compton et al., 2014; Blais et al., 2020), but they can contribute to a reduced footprint as well. For instance, as already mentioned, such efforts contribute to reduced unnecessary hospital transfers and many already have agreements in place to quickly transfer custody from the police to the hospital, both of which minimize the time PMI spend with police and thus their overall footprint. Furthermore, such efforts are likely already well more informed on the local mental health resources, as well as which resources may be especially helpful given an individual's particular situation. Research also suggests that individuals who come into contact with co-response teams have greater engagement with mental health treatment than those who have contact with frontline officers (Kisely et al., 2010). Greater treatment engagement can in turn result in reduced or even eliminated interactions with police in the future.

The Need for Continuous Evaluation

Before we conclude, we find it necessary to point out the need for continuous evaluation on each of the solutions discussed within this chapter, as well as any possible solutions that were not mentioned. The reality is that the police have long been the de facto response to PMI, both—as we have shown in this book—in a public safety capacity as well as in a crime/disorder capacity. As such, efforts which seek to minimize the footprint of the police in the lives of PMI are effectively 'new' developments and thus we currently lack a robust literature across many of the suggested solutions as to whether they are, or can, achieve this outcome. In this section we briefly discuss one practice that has been used as a means of transferring individuals that have come into contact with the police to other resources in the community. We discuss this particular practice in order to make our point for future research on footprint-reducing efforts as it has not only been widely adopted, but it has also been labelled as a 'best practice' by some government officials—a claim for which there is no evidence to support (Solicitor General, 2015).

The approach we are referring to here are known as Situation Tables or Hub Models, which we briefly discussed in the previous chapter. Increasingly common in Canada, Situation Tables often involve meetings between a myriad of community services—police, mental health services, social services, etc.—to collaboratively discuss and address cases which are understood to have an immediate risk of harm (Bhayani & Thompson, 2017; Brown & Newberry, 2015; Lamontagne, 2015). Grey literature on Situation Tables suggest that the police not only take the lead in establishing such efforts in their communities, but that they also refer the most individuals to their Situation Tables once in operation (Babayan et al., 2015; Brown & Newberry, 2015; Lamontagne, 2015; McFee & Taylor, 2014). Furthermore, of the 26 Risk Categories that are of particular interest to Situation Tables,[1] mental health is the most frequently seen category (Babayan et al., 2015). Situation Tables can thus be understood as a mechanism through which the police seek to transfer the responsibility of select PMI to other local services that may be better equipped to assist them. Indeed on the surface, Situation Tables may appear as though they are a revolutionary practice that can be used as a means to reduce the footprint of the police in the lives of some PMI. However, to-date, and in spite of its wide adoption and support from policy makers, there has not been a single, independent evaluation of Situation Tables generally, let alone an evaluation as to the impact of Situation Tables on PMI specifically. Are PMI successfully engaging with care or treatment after being the subject of a Situation Table intervention? We do not know. Do PMI who have been the subject of a Situation Table intervention have reduced or eliminated contacts with the police? We do not know. Our point here is that before supporting the mass adoption of possible solutions toward reducing the footprint of police in the lives of PMI, we must conduct rigorous evaluations to ensure that whatever solution is implemented, it achieves this particular outcome. In fact, as one of our study participants identified in the previous chapter, some PMI referred to Situation Tables can be deemed not worthy of action and thus slip through the cracks of an approach that is—at least in theory—specifically designed to help them. As such, blind adoption of practices, such as Situation Tables, will get us nowhere and—as we have seen—may even reinforce the current status quo: police as de facto responders to PMI.

---

[1] Alcohol, Drugs, Gambling, Mental Health, Suicide, Physical Health, Self-Harm, Criminal Involvement, Crime victimization, Physical Violence, Emotional Violence, Sexual Violence, Elderly Abuse, Supervision, Basic Needs, Missing School, Parenting, Housing, Poverty, Negative Peers, Antisocial/Negative Behavior, Unemployment, Missing/Runaway, Threat to Public Safety, Gangs, and Social Environment (Sanders and Langan, 2019).

Conclusions

The objective of this chapter was to bring to light some possible solutions—both outside and within policing—that could be enacted toward reducing the footprint of the police in the lives of PMI. It is important, however, that no solution is blindly put into practice without a plan to evaluate its effectiveness in terms of reducing the police footprint. In doing so, we can ensure that any enacted is achieving this desired outcome.

References

Babayan, A., Landry-Thompson, T., & Stevens, A. (2015). *Evaluation of the brant community response team initiative: Six-month report.* http://globalcommunitysafety.com/sites/default/files/brantford-six-month-evaluation.pdf

Bhayani, G., & Thompson, S. (2017). SMART on social problems: Lessons learned from a Canadian risk-based collaborative intervention model. *Policing, 11*(2), 168–184.

Blais, E., Landry, M., Elazhary, N., Carrier, S., & Savard, A.-M. (2020). Assessing the capability of a co-responding police-mental health program to connect emotionally disturbed people with community resources and decrease police use-of-force. *Journal of Experimental Criminology*, 1–25.

Brown, J., & Newberry, J. (2015). *An evaluation of the connectivity situation tables in waterloo region: Addressing risk through system collaboration.* https://cfbsjs.usask.ca/documents/research/research_papers/AnEvaluationoftheConnectivitySituationTablesinWaterlooRegion.pdf

Canada, K. E., Angell, B., & Watson, A. C. (2010). Crisis intervention teams in Chicago: Successes on the ground. *Journal of Police Crisis Negotiations, 10*(1), 86–100. https://doi.org/10.1080/15332581003792070

Charette, Y., Crocker, A. G., & Billette, I. (2011). The judicious judicial dispositions juggle: Characteristics of police interventions involving people with a mental illness. *Canadian Journal of Psychiatry, 56*(11), 677–685. https://doi.org/10.1177/070674371105601106

Children's Mental Health Ontario. (2020). *Kids can't wait: 2020 report on wait lists and wait times for child and youth mental health care in Ontario.* https://cmho.org/wp-content/uploads/CMHO-Report-WaitTimes-2020.pdf

Compton, M. T., Bakeman, R., Broussard, B., Hankerson-Dyson, D., Husbands, L., Krishan, S., ... Watson, A. C. (2014). The police-based crisis intervention team (CIT) Model: II. effects on level of force and resolution, referral, and arrest. *Psychiatric Services, 65*(4), 523–529.

Fahim, C., Semovski, V., & Younger, J. (2016). The Hamilton mobile crisis rapid response team: A first-responder mental health service. *Psychiatric Services, 67*(8), 929. https://doi.org/10.1176/appi.ps.670802

Goldner, E. M., Jones, W., & Fang, M. L. (2011). Access to and waiting time for psychiatrist services in a Canadian urban area: A study in real time. *The Canadian Journal of Psychiatry, 56*(8), 474–480. https://doi.org/10.1177/070674371105600805

Harris, K. M., & Edlund, M. J. (2005). Use of mental health care and substance abuse treatment among adults with co-occurring disorders. *Psychiatric Services, 56*(8), 954–959.

HealthIM. (n.d.) *HealthIM.* https://healthim.com/

Hirdes, J., van Everdingen, C., Ferris, J., Franco-Martin, M., Fries, B., et al. (2019). The interRAI suite of mental health assessment instruments: An integrated system for the continuum of care. *Frontiers in Psychiatry, 10*, 926–956.

References

Hodgkinson, T. K., & Andresen, M. A. (2019). Understanding the spatial patterns of police activity and mental health in a Canadian city. *Journal of Contemporary Criminal Justice, 35*(2), 221–240. https://doi.org/10.1177/1043986219842014

Hoffman, R., Hirdes, J., Brown, G., Dubin, J., & Barbaree, H. (2016). The use of a brief mental health screener to enhance the ability of police officers to identify persons with serious mental disorders. *International Journal of Law and Psychiatry, 47*(1), 28–35.

Huey, L., & Broll, R. (2018). *Becoming strong: Impoverished women and the struggle to overcome violence.* University of Toronto Press.

Iacobucci, F. (2014). *Police encounters with people in crisis.* Toronto Police Service.

Kirst, M., Zerger, S., Misir, V., Hwang, S., & Stergiopoulos, V. (2015). The impact of a Housing First randomized controlled trial on substance use problems among homeless individuals with mental illness. *Drug and Alcohol Dependence, 146,* 24–29.

Kisely, S., Campbell, L. A., Peddle, S., Hare, S., Pyche, M., Spicer, D., & Moore, B. (2010). A controlled before-and-after evaluation of a mobile crisis partnership between mental health and police services in Nova Scotia. *Canadian Journal of Psychiatry, 55*(10), 662–668. https://doi.org/10.1177/070674371005501005

Koziarski, J. (2020). Examining the spatial concentration of mental health calls for police service in a small city. *Policing: A Journal of Policy and Practice,* 1–18. https://doi.org/10.1093/police/paaa093

Koziarski, J., O'Connor, C., & Frederick, T. (2020). Policing mental health: The composition and perceived challenges of co-response teams and crisis intervention teams in the Canadian context. *Police Practice and Research, 22*(1), 1–19.

Lamb, H., Weinberger, L., & DeCuir, W. (2002). The police and mental health. *Psychiatric Services, 53*(10), 1266–1271.

Lamb, R. H., & Bachrach, L. L. (2001). Some perspective on deinstitutionalization. *Psychiatric Services, 52*(8), 1039–1045.

Lamontagne, E. (2015). Rapid mobilization table data analysis. https://cfbsjs.usask.ca/documents/research/research_papers/RMTDataAnalysisReport.pdf

Lurie, S. (2014). Why can't Canada spend more on mental health? *Health, 6,* 684–690. https://doi.org/10.4236/health.2014.68089

Markowitz, F. E. (2011). Mental illness, crime, and violence: Risk, context, and social control. *Aggression and Violent Behavior, 16*(1), 36–44. https://doi.org/10.1016/j.avb.2010.10.003

McFee, D., & Taylor, N. (2014). *The prince albert hub and the emergence of collaborative risk-driven community safety.* https://cfbsjs.usask.ca/documents/research/research_papers/ChangeAndInnovationInCanadianPolicing.pdf

Padgett, D. K., Stanhope, V., Henwood, B. F., et al. (2011). Substance use outcomes among homeless clients with serious mental illness: Comparing housing first with treatment first programs. *Community Mental Health Journal, 47,* 227–232. https://doi.org/10.1007/s10597-009-9283-7

Ratcliffe, J. H. (2021). Policing and public health calls for service in Philadelphia. *Crime Science,* 1–6. https://doi.org/10.1186/s40163-021-00141-0

Sanders, C. B. & Langan, D. (2019) New public management and the extension of police control: community safety and security networks in Canada. *Policing and Society, 29*(5), 566–578. https://doi.org/10.1080/10439463.2018.1427744.

Schulenberg, J. (2016). Police decision-making in the gray zone: The dynamics of police–citizen encounters with mentally ill persons. *Criminal Justice and Behavior, 43*(4), 459–482.

Semple, T., Tomlin, M., Bennell, C., & Jenkins, B. (2020). An evaluation of a community - based mobile crisis intervention team in a small Canadian police service. *Community Mental Health Journal.* https://doi.org/10.1007/s10597-020-00683-8

Shore, K., & Lavoie, J. (2019). Exploring mental health-related calls for police service: A Canadian study of police officers as 'frontline mental health workers'. *Policing: A Journal of Policy and Practice, 13*(2), 157–171.

Solicitor General. (2015). *Public safety Canada – 2nd summit on the economics of policing and community safety.* https://news.ontario.ca/en/speech/31960/public-safety-canada%2D%2D-2nd-summit-on-the-economics-of-policing-community-safety

Steadman, H. J., Stainbrook, K. A., Griffin, P., Draine, J., Dupont, R., & Horey, C. (2001). A specialized crisis response site as a core element of police-based diversion programs. *Psychiatric Services, 52*(2), 219–222. https://doi.org/10.1176/appi.ps.52.2.219

Teplin, L., & Pruett, N. (1992). Police as streetcorner psychiatrist: Managing the mentally ill. *International Journal of Law and Psychiatry, 15*(2), 139–156.

Vaughan, A. D., Hewitt, A. N., Andresen, M. A., & Brantingham, P. L. (2016). Exploring the role of the environmental context in the spatial distribution of calls-for-service associated with emotionally disturbed persons. *Policing, 10*(2), 121–133. https://doi.org/10.1093/police/pav040

Vaughan, A. D., Ly, M., Andresen, M. A., Wuschke, K., Hodgkinson, T., & Campbell, A. (2018). Concentrations and specialization of mental health–related calls for police service. *Victims and Offenders, 13*(8), 1153–1170. https://doi.org/10.1080/15564886.2018.1512539

Watson, A., & Wood, J. D. (2017). Everyday police work during mental health encounters: A study of call resolutions in Chicago and their implications for diversion. *Behavioral Sciences & the Law, 35*(5–6), 442–455.

Wells, W., & Schafer, J. (2006). Officer perceptions of police responses to persons with a mental illness. *Policing: An International Journal of Police Strategies & Management, 29*(4), 578–601.

White Bird Clinic. (2020). *What is CAHOOTS?* https://whitebirdclinic.org/what-is-cahoots/

White, C., & Goldberg, V. (2018). Hot spots of mental health crises: A look at the concentration of mental health calls and future directions for policing. *Policing: An International Journal, 41*(3), 401–414. https://doi.org/10.1108/PIJPSM-12-2017-0155

White, C., & Weisburd, D. (2017). A co-responder model for policing mental health problems at crime hot spots: Findings from a pilot project. *Policing: A Journal of Policy and Practice, 12*(2), 194–209.

Appendix: The Studies

A central focus of the data collected from both studies upon which we rely was the use of discretion in frontline police decision-making.

Data Collection

As noted, data used here was collected through two separate studies in two Canadian cities. Both studies were approved by University research ethics board[1] and all research was conducted in accordance with Canadian Tri-Council guidelines for executing research involving human participants.

Site 1

The first study combined systematic social observation with interviews and analysis of calls for service data to examine policing of antisocial behaviour. This study produced detailed field notes supplemented with data from in-depth qualitative interviews conducted with 16 participants.[2] Field notes captured events occurring during 74 police ride-alongs, which comprised approximately 637 h of

---

[1] As other researchers have observed, the ability to collect data through field-based observations is a feat that is becoming increasingly more difficult due to reluctance by University ethics boards to approve this type of work (Haggerty 2004), as well as increased unwillingness by many police organizations (Schulenberg 2014).

[2] As these interviews were more narrowly focused on issues related to youth in conflict with the law, we opted not to rely on this data source.

© The Author(s), under exclusive license to Springer Nature Switzerland AG 2022
L. Huey et al., *Policing Mental Health*, SpringerBriefs in Criminology,
https://doi.org/10.1007/978-3-030-94313-4

observations. In total, 406 police-citizen encounters with 568 individuals were documented during the study period.

All fieldwork for this project was undertaken by one of the authors. Ride-alongs were conducted with patrol officers across all divisions during the period of November 2011 to June 2012 and data was collected on both the early (1:30–11:30 p.m.) and late afternoon shift (5:00 p.m.–3:00 a.m.) from Thursday to Sunday. Divisions and platoons were randomly selected; however, which officers the researcher rode with was at the sole discretion of the area Staff-Sergeant. Prior to each shift, the researcher brought specific forms, termed a 'ride-along sheet' which were intended to capture relevant details about the 'encounter' and 'citizen characteristics'. For example, information about the actions, attitudes, beliefs, and behaviours of individuals in the following roles was observed and recorded: 'complainant/victim', 'suspect/person of interest', 'disputant/subject', 'helpless person/check wellbeing', and 'witness', among others. Encounter characteristics included, among other details: 'type of call for service', 'particulars of the encounter', 'police actions', and 'background information'. Each ride-along sheet was assigned an identifying number, as was each encounter. Forms were filled out as soon after an encounter as was practicable, and all information related to an encounter was input within 8–12 h following a ride-along.

The site in which this research was conducted is a region comprised of three urban and two rural areas. One of those urban areas is best described as an 'university town', a home to some 50,000 undergraduate and postgraduate students. The total population of this region at the time of this study was approximately 536,793 individuals, with a crime rate of 5264 per 100,000 population.

Site 2

The second study—conducted from 2015 to 2016—similarly employed systematic social observation in field-based settings. Observations were conducted during 36 ride-alongs with patrol officers. Two trained observers accompanied frontline personnel on their shifts. And, as with the previous study, were granted access to accompany and observe officers during the bulk of encounters.[3] Following a call for service or other 'encounter', an observation sheet was filled out by the field researcher—typically, in the patrol car when time officers were occupied with paperwork or other tasks. To ensure a degree of reliability in recorded observations, researchers also used this time to query officers about the event and, in some instances, asked officers to review notes taken for accuracy. These information sheets were then input into computerized field notes—with extra description added

---

[3] The only exceptions were a handful of instances, where for safety reasons, researchers were requested to stay in the patrol vehicle or to otherwise stay at a distance from an encounter.

based on additional field observations—as soon as practicable by the researcher (usually within 24 h).

These officers work within a small city in southwestern Ontario that is principally noted for its tourism. Although a significant tourist site, it is located within a predominately agricultural area of the province with some manufacturing and a satellite campus of a major university. The population here is just under 40,000 citizens, and the crime rate is 5290 per 100,000.

References

Schulenberg, J. L. (2014). Systematic social observation of police decision-making: The process, logistics, and challenges in a Canadian context. *Quality & Quantity: International Journal of Methodology*, 48, 297–315. https://doi.org/10.1007/s11135-012-9769-1.

Haggerty, K.D. (2004). Ethics Creep: Governing Social Science Research in the Name of Ethics. *Qualitative Sociology*, 27, 391–414. https://doi.org/10.1023/B:QUAS.0000049239.15922.a3.

Index

A
Allegations, 1
Antisocial behaviour, 6
Attempt suicide, 20
Attention Deficit Disorder, 34

C
Calling the cops, 4
Call type code, 7
Canadian police services, 5, 10
Community, 49, 50
Community-based mental health resources, 53
Community death notifications, 24
Computerized field notes, 60
Continuous evaluation, 54, 55
Crime, 3, 4, 10
Crime/disorder domains, 49
Crime prevention
    complainant calls, 29, 30
    criminal justice response, 27
    criminal suspects, 32–35
    decision-making, 27
    disturbance/disorderly conduct, 31, 32
    law enforcement orientation, 27
    police interactions, 27
    potential threats, 35, 36
    potential victims/harm, 31
    public safety-related, 36
    victimization calls, 28, 29
Crime response, 10
Criminal justice system, 52
Criminal victimization, 28
Crisis Intervention Teams (CIT), 54

D
Death notifications, 23
Defund the police, 49
De-institutionalization, 1
Demand changes, 49
Depression, 34
Disorder, 3, 4, 10, 27
Driving-related complaints, 23
Drug
    Abuse Resistance Education (D.A.R.E.), 2
Drug use, 2, 3

E
Emergency Response Unit (ERU), 36
Encounter, 60
Encounter 23, 23, 24
Encounter 71, 21
Encounter 99, 21
Encounter 106, 18
Encounter 134, 22, 23
Encounter 138, 19
Encounter 240, 20
Encounter 249, 22
Encounter 280, 17
Encounter 335, 20
Encounter 367, 16
Encounter characteristics, 60
Ethnicity-based data, 9, 10

F
Family and Children Services, 34
Field notes, 6, 7, 59

Flag M, 6
Follow-up calls, 15, 23, 24

H
Harm, 15, 16, 19, 24
Healthcare professionals, 52
Homelessness and substance use, 51
Hospital- and community-based mental health care, 50

I
Individual-/family-level approaches, 51
interRAI Brief Mental Health Screener, 5

M
Mental health, 3
    Canadian police services, 5
    police property, 1
    screener, 5
Mental Health Act (MHA), 16, 17, 22–24, 29, 32, 43–44, 53
Mental health apprehensions, 15–18
Mental health care, 50, 51
Mental health issues
    anxiety issues, 40
    disorders, 40
    family dysfunction, 40
    interview data, 39
    mental illness, 40
    oppositional defiance disorder, 40
    police officers, 39
        criminal/activity, 43
        criminal conduct, 44
        police protocols, 45
        police services, 44
        psychiatric facilities, 43
        public policy, 43
        research, 45
    police property
        drugs and self-harming, 41
        free taxi service, 41
        healthcare system, 41
        interview, 42
        mental health-related calls, 41
        police agencies, 40
        police gatekeeping function, 42
        police role, 43
        private conversation, 42
        risk factors, 42
        violence, 41
    police resources, 39
    research field, 39
Mental health legislation, 1, 53
Mental health-related calls police attend, 5
Mental health system, 51
Mental illness, 5, 33, 35, 51
Metropolitan Police Act, 3
Missing person' call, 15, 17, 18
Mobile Crisis Unit, 29
Mobile mental health application, 5

N
Narcotics, 2
9-1-1 calls, 17, 19–24
Notifications, 18
Not social workers, 4

O
Order maintenance, 2–4

P
Persons with mental illness (PMI), 1, 3, 4, 7–11
Police decision-making, 59
Police intervention, 34
Police involvement, 6, 9, 17, 24
Police mobilization, 3–4
Police property, 1–4, 6, 49, 50
Police RMS, 6, 8, 10
Police role, 16, 17, 24
Policing, 10
    antisocial behaviour, 6
    drug war, 2
    era of innovation, 3
    interactions, 15
    'one-size-fits-all' model, 3
    police property, 2
Public policing, 49
Public safety, 3, 4, 10, 15, 24, 49

R
Record management systems (RMS), 6, 8, 10
Reform, 49
Ride-along, 60
Ride-along sheet, 60

S
Safety, 17, 19
Situation Table intervention, 55
Skid-row, 2, 3
Social behaviours, 4
Social workers, 52
Social work role, 4

Solutions, 50, 54–56
Substance use, 2, 3, 5, 10, 51
Sudden death, 22–24
Suicide, 20–23
Suicide attempts, 19, 22
Suicide-related calls, 22
Systematic social observation, 6, 59, 60

T
Traffic-related incident, 49
24/7 service providers, 4

U
Unfortunate reality, 10
Uniform Crime Reporting (UCR) data, 10
University town, 60

V
Vice crimes, 2

W
Wellness checks, 15, 19, 20

GPSR Compliance

The European Union's (EU) General Product Safety Regulation (GPSR) is a set of rules that requires consumer products to be safe and our obligations to ensure this.

If you have any concerns about our products, you can contact us on

ProductSafety@springernature.com

In case Publisher is established outside the EU, the EU authorized representative is:

Springer Nature Customer Service Center GmbH
Europaplatz 3
69115 Heidelberg, Germany